Patient–Provider Communications: Caring to Listen

Valerie A. Hart, EdD, APRN, PMHCNS
Associate Professor of Nursing, University of Southern Maine
Private Psychotherapy Practice
Portland, Maine

JONES AND BARTLETT PUBLISHERS
Sudbury, Massachusetts
BOSTON   TORONTO   LONDON   SINGAPORE

World Headquarters

Jones and Bartlett Publishers	Jones and Bartlett Publishers	Jones and Bartlett Publishers
40 Tall Pine Drive	Canada	International
Sudbury, MA 01776	6339 Ormindale Way	Barb House, Barb Mews
978-443-5000	Mississauga, Ontario L5V 1J2	London W6 7PA
info@jbpub.com	Canada	United Kingdom
www.jbpub.com		

Jones and Bartlett's books and products are available through most bookstores and online booksellers. To contact Jones and Bartlett Publishers directly, call 800-832-0034, fax 978-443-8000, or visit our website, www.jbpub.com.

Substantial discounts on bulk quantities of Jones and Bartlett's publications are available to corporations, professional associations, and other qualified organizations. For details and specific discount information, contact the special sales department at Jones and Bartlett via the above contact information or send an email to specialsales@jbpub.com.

The authors, editors, and publisher have made every effort to provide accurate information. However, they are not responsible for errors, omissions, or for any outcomes related to the use of the contents of this book and take no responsibility for the use of the products and procedures described. Treatments and side effects described in this book may not be applicable to all people; likewise, some people may require a dose or experience a side effect that is not described herein. Drugs and medical devices are discussed that may have limited availability controlled by the Food and Drug Administration (FDA) for use only in a research study or clinical trial. Research, clinical practice, and government regulations often change the accepted standard in this field. When consideration is being given to use of any drug in the clinical setting, the health care provider or reader is responsible for determining FDA status of the drug, reading the package insert, and reviewing prescribing information for the most up-to-date recommendations on dose, precautions, and contraindications, and determining the appropriate usage for the product. This is especially important in the case of drugs that are new or seldom used.

Production Credits
Publisher: Kevin Sullivan
Acquisitions Editor: Emily Ekle
Acquisitions Editor: Amy Sibley
Editorial Assistant: Rachel Shuster
Production Editor: Amanda Clerkin
Marketing Manager: Rebecca Wasley
V.P., Manufacturing and Inventory Control: Therese Connell
Composition: DDC/ASI
Cover Design: Scott Moden
Cover Image: © Uguntina/Shutterstock, Inc.
Printing and Binding: Malloy, Inc.
Cover Printing: Malloy, Inc.

Library of Congress Cataloging-in-Publication Data
Hart, Valerie, 1950-
  Patient-provider communications : caring to listen / Valerie A. Hart.
    p. ; cm.
Includes bibliographical references and index.
ISBN-13: 978-0-7637-6169-1 (alk. paper)
ISBN-10: 0-7637-6169-9 (alk. paper)
1. Nurse and patient. 2. Communication in medicine. I. Title.
[DNLM: 1. Nurse-Patient Relations. 2. Communication. WY 87 H325p 2010]
RT86.3.H37 2010
610.7306′9—dc22   2009018670

6048

Printed in United States of America
13 12 11 10 09   10 9 8 7 6 5 4 3 2 1

Dedication

To all my very patient, understanding, and tolerant family and friends who were so very supportive and understanding of my time limitations while I "worked on the book," my thanks and love. In particular, my parents, John and Elizabeth Hart; my beautiful and loving children, John and Paige, who have always been my greatest inspiration; my loving partner, Dave Morrison; my generous contributors whose expertise I appreciate; and, of course, all of my students, past, present, and future, who were the driving force behind this project and may benefit from the work. Finally, for all patients who deserve caring providers who can communicate effectively in order to deliver expert care.

Contents

Contributors

Valerie A. Hart, EdD, APRN, PMHCNS
Associate Professor of Nursing
University of Southern Maine
Private Psychotherapy Practice
Portland, Maine

Elcha Shain Buckman, ARNP-CS/ APRN-CS, BC (Ret.)
Adjunct Professor
Nova Southeastern University
Davie, Florida
Private Practice
Fort Lauderdale, Florida, and
    Boston, Massachusetts

Ann M. McPhee, MS, RN, MSB
Nursing Director, Outpatient
    Department
Interim Nursing Director
Barbara Bush Children's Hospital-
    Maine Medical Center
Portland, Maine

L. Susan Yetter, PhD, APRN, PMH-NP, CS
Assistant Professor
College of Nursing and Health
    Professions
University of Southern Maine
Portland, Maine

Introduction

Valerie A. Hart

Over 30 years ago, Marlene Kramer coined the term *reality shock* to describe the challenges facing new nurses as they wrestled with the values and procedures that increasingly are viewed as idealistic once in the working environment (Kramer, 1974). It can be safely argued that the pressures have increased since the time that this concept was described. Both undergraduate and graduate programs in nursing stress a holistic framework in which to evaluate patients and families and in which to provide patient care. This framework is one way that the profession of nursing differentiates itself from other healthcare disciplines. The harsh realities of the workplace, including both in-patient care in large institutions as well as out-patient clinics and practices, is often based on the medical model of patient care and a bureaucratic organizational model. This creates a serious challenge to the demands of holism, in considering psychosocial aspects of a patient's experience when performing an assessment and in providing care. The profession of nursing has long been involved in caring for and talking to patients. It was the specialty of psychiatric–mental health nursing that led the way in the development of concepts related to nurse–patient relationships and communication. Chapter 1 is a close examination of the theories that served to guide early nursing theorists and will inform today's clinician when communicating with patients and families. These theorists were inspired by philosophers, theologians, psychologists, and other mental health giants. Beyond understanding theories of communication this text utilizes several other theories, including those related to reflective practice and the professional development of novice to expert. Utilizing the tenets of reflective practice, both communication exercises and journaling exercises are included in each chapter. Only by increasing self-awareness can a clinician be truly effective with patients and develop the capacity to have a lengthy career in such a challenging field as health care. In addition, this book explores the overarching frame of working with patients in patient- and family-centered care. This framework requires a certain type of clinician and a very specific type of communication.

Health care today is clearly in trouble, and healthcare providers are being asked to deliver quality care despite the demands of the setting in which they work, third-party payers, the constraints of managed care, and, most importantly, patients and their families. Revamping the nation's healthcare system is a topic that caught the attention of candidates for the presidential election of 2008. The question of health care as a right or privilege continues to be debated across the United States, and the ultimate national consensus regarding this question will transform the future of health care for decades to come. Chapter 2 examines issues related to communication in the light of the present healthcare environment. With the increasing pressure for more efficient and cost-effective health care, providers are faced with balancing the business side of their work with the importance of their relationships with patients. They must struggle to sustain the satisfaction derived from providing the kind of care they learned was possible in their educational programs or that originally brought them to the field.

While the relationship between communication and health outcomes is rarely researched, some findings about this topic would seem to indicate that what patients and quality assurance experts see as important can differ. For example, while much of the research on cancer communications focuses on patients' recall of recommendations and whether follow-through occurs, patients are understandably most interested in their health, survival, and quality of life (Epstein & Street, 2007). It seems even when trying to improve communication with patients we may be guilty of miscommunication. Another study of recorded conversations between patients and their oncologist (Pollak et al., 2007) found patterns of cutting patients off when the emotional aspects of cancer were voiced by patients. The researchers call for additional training in recognizing and responding to the emotional needs of patients. It is in this spirit that Chapters 3 and 4 examine the specifics of what it means to be an effective communicator with patients. This includes the ability to listen, truly listen, to our patients and families. In addition, challenging issues such as the professional role versus one's personal life will be examined in light of patient communications. In Chapter 3 issues of self disclosure and boundaries will be explored in an attempt to guide the clinician in developing the skills required for therapeutic communication. One of the most complex concepts is that of the difference between a personal and a professional relationship and the communication skills that are inherent in the latter.

Chapter 5 explores specific issues related to communicating with patients across the life span, describing communication strategies with children, adolescents, and elders. One of the most daunting clinical encounters is one that consists of communicating bad news to a patient or family member. There is clearly an art and a science to this communication that can guide the clinician. Chapter 6 examines difficult conversations of a wide variety and offers clues for the clinician in these most challenging interactions. In Chapter 7, issues related to the importance of cultural sensitivity in relationship to patient communication are discussed.

Consumers of health care have consistently placed the relationship with their healthcare provider high in the priority list of what they seek. Patient satisfaction surveys are here to stay and they demand that clinicians have the skills to effectively communicate. Clinicians need to talk to their patients about both routine and difficult healthcare issues. Popular magazines today offer tips on how to get better care when visiting a healthcare provider, considering the brief amount of time allotted for a clinical visit. One such article in *Glamour's* health section (2007) advises patients to bring up the important issues first, using the template of *the four w's* (when it began, what it feels like, what makes it better, and what makes it worse); cutting off any small talk when the provider talks about themselves; and asking to do a summary of what was decided before exiting the room. While I applaud the educational aspect of the article, which can prepare patients to use their time efficiently, the fact that there is a need for such a primer is disturbing. New nursing graduates are expected to practice in a safe manner, supervise other staff, communicate effectively with patients and families, be technically proficient in carrying out procedures, and complete assignments in an appropriate time frame. These requirements are often spelled out by the various boards of nursing in the state in which a new graduate is licensed. It can be argued that the majority of these expectations require the skills of communication. In most health-related graduate programs hundreds of hours are spent on providing student practice focused on technical proficiency, which is a reasonable requirement. However, much less time, if any, is devoted to assuring that the future healthcare provider is a master communicator. On both the graduate and undergraduate level there is a requirement for nurses to work alongside other healthcare providers in a collaborative manner. Chapter 8 examines the issue of interdisciplinary communications in health care.

In an article on role discrepancy, Takase, Maude, and Manias (2006) studied nurses' perceptions of the differences between ideal and actual nursing roles and related these differences to the nurses' length of experience. They found that, while nurses with more clinical experience rated their ideal and actual roles more positively than those with less experience, *both* reportedly experienced the same degree of role discrepancy in certain areas. These included organizational decision-making and providing patient education. The authors conclude that nursing cannot resolve role discrepancy simply by increasing the length of clinicals but, rather, educators need to assist students in actualizing their ideal views of practice in today's healthcare environment.

It has been suggested that in recent years nursing has focused more on building a scientific foundation for practice and there has been less attention to the art of nursing, which is demonstrated by the concept of caring (Jansen, 2006). It is interesting how often the words as used together, nursing and caring. Consider critical care nursing, home healthcare nursing, nursing home care, or simply nursing care. In addition, when we consider the places nurses work, we find care to be a prominent component, such as home care, renal care, postoperative care, and out-patient care. And the world of healthcare reimbursement has adopted the term when devising the concept of managed care.

There is much interest in the ethics of caring in nursing (Kuhse, Singer, Rickard, Cannold, & van Dyk, 1997). While tracing the nurse–physician relationship from servant to patient advocate, the authors identify ethical dilemmas along the way. They explore the ethics of care and challenge others in the field of ethics while underscoring the importance of communication skills for today's healthcare provider. Due to the pace of care delivery and acuity of patients, advanced communication skills are even more important than in the past. Among the recommendations are provision of dispositional care, meaning "a willingness and openness to apprehend the health-related reality of the other," recognizing patients as particular others having special needs, beliefs, and desires. This approach can also serve as a useful corrective to a tendency under the medical model to treat patients predominantly as "malfunctioning organisms" (Kuhse et al. 1997, p. 150). In the case of patient communication, the practice involves finding one's own words in a variety of clinical situations, learning by making mistakes, and learning by receiving feedback from the recipient of their communication messages.

Specific issues related to advanced practice are addressed in Chapter 9, including guidance from the business world. Today's health care has become more of a business model and, therefore, providers need to be familiar with the opportunities and challenges represented by this model.

Chapter 10 introduces the concept of peer groups. Because advanced practice nurses are still either pioneering new roles or working in an isolated environment, the value of forming or joining a peer group is explored. The author's experience in creating a structure for running a successful peer group is also described.

My experience in teaching communication skills to future nurse clinicians, nurse practitioners, midwives, administrators, and educators has convinced me that it is only by role playing and self-evaluation and reflection that these skills develop to the point of transferring from the classroom to the actual clinical setting. It is not enough to have a theoretical understanding of the use of silence, one must practice this skill and work through the discomfort that a novice experiences in order to place it in the toolkit of clinical strategies when in the middle of a patient interaction. As a result, this text offers current research in the area of patient–provider communications and provides suggestions for transferring theory into practice. It facilitates reflective awareness and teaches a framework for ongoing professional growth for the advanced practice nurse. In addition to providing growth for the reader in the area of communication application in the clinical setting, the text offers the latest information on communication with children, adolescents, elders, and those with alcohol and drug abuse issues. The topic of interdisciplinary communication is addressed along with current issues in health care that impact provider–patient communications. Specific issues related to advance practice nursing are addressed in Chapter 9, including a primer on incorporating business principles and practices into one's professional practice.

The communication exercises in this text are meant to be done in pairs or as a trio and should be accompanied by analysis and discussion by students and their professors. Because the audience is at the graduate level they will include specific areas that take into account where advanced healthcare practitioners practice. It assumes a beginning knowledge of communication theory pertinent to the healthcare environment.

The journaling exercises are meant to deepen student self-awareness of the issues related to patient communication. In order to be an effective clinician one must be highly self-aware and these assignments are intended to facilitate this work. Students may share these insights with peers and they may be used in the classroom as a foundation for seminar discussions. Used in conjunction with the communication exercises the journaling assignments will assist the student in integrating communication theory and form a solid foundation for clinical practice. Novice and seasoned, advanced practice nurses, as well as healthcare providers in other disciplines, will benefit from taking a closer look at their particular communication strengths and weaknesses. Only by finding the words ourselves can we become proficient in patient communications. It is not enough to read about communication theory, it must be put into practice and then practiced some more. My hope is that this text will start this journey for clinicians who have a basic knowledge in this area and will continue their professional development in the intriguing area of patient–provider communications. It is the ability to communicate and form deeply satisfying relationships with our patients and their families that are the best antidote against such highly demanding and yet rewarding work.

REFERENCES

Epstein, R., & Street, R. (2007). *Patient-centered communication in cancer care.* Publication 07-6225. Bethesda, MD: National Institutes of Health.

Get a better checkup! (2007, November). *Glamour*, p. 130.

Kuhse, H. (1997). *Caring: Nurses, women and ethics.* Malden, MA: Blackwell.

Jansen, M. P. (2006). Advanced practice within a nursing paradigm. In M. P. Jansen, & M. Zwygart-Stauffacher (Eds.), *Advanced practice nursing: Core concepts for professional role development* (3rd ed.). New York: Springer.

Kramer, M. (1974). *Reality shock: Why nurses leave nursing.* St. Louis, MO: Mosby.

Kuhse, H., Singer, P., Rickard, M., Cannold, L., & van Dyk, J. (1997). Partial and impartial ethical reasoning in health care professionals. *Journal of Medical Ethics, 23*(4), 226–232.

Pollak, K., Jeffreys, A. R., Alexander, S. A., Olsen, S., Abernethy, M., Sugg, A., et al. (2007). Oncologist communication about emotion during visits with patients with advanced cancer. *Journal of Clinical Oncology, 57,* 48–52.

Takase, M., Maude, P., & Manias, E. (2006). Role discrepancy: is it a common problem among nurses? *Journal of Advanced Nursing, 54*(6), 751–759.

SUGGESTED READINGS

Benner, P. (2000). *From novice to expert: Excellence and power in clinical nursing practice.* Upper Saddle River, NJ: Prentice Hall.

Buber, M. (1970). *I and thou* (Kaufmann trans.). New York: Charles Scribner's Sons.

CHAPTER 1

Communication and Nursing: Historical Roots and Related Theory

Valerie A. Hart

Practice helps to impress and retain in the memory the knowledge obtained by theory, otherwise forgotten without the practical application. Any one who has been ill knows that the height of good nursing consists principally in what is done for the patient's comfort, outside of the regular orders. A theoretical nurse performs her duty in a perfunctory manner, and may carry out the doctor's orders to the letter; but the patient recognizes there is something lacking, and we know that it is the skilled touch, the deft handling, the keenness to detect changes and symptoms, the ready tact, the patience, the power of controlling her feelings and temper, self-reliance, the kindly sympathy for the sorrowing, and the peculiar power of soothing suffering which can be acquired only by much practice; and a nurse without these attributes, despite her wide theoretic knowledge and teaching, will never be a successful one (Brennan, 2006, p. 191).

In this chapter, the early roots and influences of communications and nursing will be explored. In addition to acknowledging the contributions of those concerned with the subject of patient communication, this text primarily utilizes theories related to patient-centered care, novice to expert development, and reflective practice. These theories will be explored and will form the foundation for the focus of communication practice for the advanced practice nurse. The text will build on basic communication theory and encourage the reader to hone their skills in this area.

Tracing the role and importance of communication theory and practice in nursing requires an amount of speculation and reliance on early nursing curriculum. In order to understand the place of communication theory in nursing practice, we must look to the past and fully explore the early nursing pioneers and those theorists who influenced them. It is also important to remember that nursing, for many decades, was attempting to carve out a clear definition of itself, a scope of

1

practice in order to take its place as a true profession. Many nursing programs today give only a brief allotment of time to the subject of nursing history. While nursing history, once was a staple in the nursing curriculum as a way to acculturate the new student, over time has been shed and replaced by other content.

The American Association for the History of Nursing (AAHN) has developed a position statement regarding the importance of including nursing history in the curriculum in order to prepare nurses for the 21st century. AAHN recommends that nursing history be included in both undergraduate and graduate curricula and that a separate course in nursing history be part of any doctoral program in nursing (AAHN, 2001). By examining the historical roots of the concepts of patient–provider relationships, and what constitutes nursing care, we can clearly explore the topic of provider communications with patients and families. Without the proper backdrop it might seem like a new idea when, in fact, it has been emphasized by nursing educators and practitioners since the first nurse ministered to the first patient.

EARLY NURSING EDUCATION

Initially, nursing education was based on the apprentice model of education and was designed to meet the service needs of the hospital with which the school was affiliated (Box 1-1). Although not all schools of nursing were affiliated with hospitals, this was certainly the template developed by Florence Nightingale

Box 1-1   Early Development of Nursing Education

1893, formation of The National League for Nursing Education
1917, release of the first standard curriculum for schools of nursing
1918, Goldmark Report, assessing nursing education
1928, *Nurses, Patients, and Pocketbooks* published
1934, *Nursing Schools Today and Tomorrow* published
1936, publication of NLNE *Essentials of a Good School of Nursing* (Effie Taylor, president)
1937, revision of NLNE's curriculum guide

and adopted in the United States. Although there was some variation in early nursing curricula, it is safe to assume that the emphasis was on practical work and service. A typical example is the 1918 curriculum from the University of Texas School of Nursing, the oldest nursing school in Texas and one of the oldest in the Southwest. Established in 1890 as the John Sealy Hospital Training School of Nurses, it was originally organized as an independent school under a board of lay managers. The didactic classroom requirements were as follows (Pope, 1937):

First Year:
　　Anatomy and Physiology: 30 hours
　　Fever Nursing: 12 hours
　　Theory of Nursing: 12 hours
　　Bacteriology: 14 hours
　　Preventative Medicine: 14 hours
　　Materia Medica: 15 hours

Second Year:
　　Surgical Nursing: 14 hours
　　Medical Nursing: 10 hours
　　Gynecological Nursing: 15 hours
　　Obstetrical Nursing: 15 hours
　　Diatetics:15 hours
　　Invalid Cookery: 40 hours

Third Year:
　　Pediatric Nursing: 8 hours
　　Eye, Ear, Nose, and Throat: 8 hours
　　Mental and Nervous Disease: 6 hours
　　Theory of Nursing: 20 hours
　　Ethics: 6 hours
　　Massage: 32 hours.

Total for Three Years: 314 hours

　　We cannot know for certain what was included in a lecture on the "Theory of Nursing," and it is possible that the topic of patient communication was squeezed into the brief time allocated for "Mental and Nervous Disease." But it is more likely that very little time was devoted to the topic of patient communication. This early curriculum is a typical example of what followed from the 1917 release of the first Standard Curriculum for Schools of Nursing, developed by the National League for Nursing Education. This organization, formed in 1893, during the Chicago World's Fair, was originally the American Society of

Superintendents of Training Schools for Nurses. From its inception, the association made its principal objective the "establishment and maintenance of a universal standard of training." In 1912 the society was renamed the National League for Nursing Education (NLNE).

It was not until after World War I and the influenza pandemic had receded that nursing leaders would take stock of the state of nursing education in the United States. In 1918, a 5-year study funded by the Rockefeller Foundation was initiated and aimed to assess the current condition of nursing education in the United States. Commonly referred to as the Goldmark Report (a member of the committee), this study highlighted the many weaknesses of the apprentice model of nursing education (Dolan, 1983). The Goldmark Report was critical of the relationship schools had with hospitals, the quality of faculty and overall education, and made strong recommendations for change. Unlike the Flexner Report, the equivalent study of medical schools, this report was not made public and, even if some schools closed as a result, the vast majority did not and nothing changed in regard to the model of nursing education. Overall, the sharp criticism in the Goldmark Report did little to make changes in how nursing education was delivered, how schools were organized, or what the nursing curriculum looked like. The financial ties that nursing schools had to hospitals were simply too strong and, thus, the incentive to keep doing business as usual prevailed. Instead of reform, more studies of nursing followed, including *Nurses, Patients and Pocketbooks* (1928) and *Nursing Schools Today and Tomorrow* (1934), both instigated by the American Nurses Association (ANA). Again, the findings reported serious shortcomings on the part of faculty preparation as well as the actual educational programs. Perhaps as a way of addressing these concerns, the NLNE published a specific guide in 1936, *Essentials of a Good School of Nursing*. This guide provided the scaffolding for what was "essential" in nursing and, therefore, nursing curricula. It is interesting to note that among the eight guidelines regarding what a professional nurse should know, number four was:

All professional nurses should be able to apply, in nursing situations, those principles of mental hygiene which make for a better understanding of the psychological factor in illness (National League for Nursing [NLN], 1936).

This criterion may be interpreted as an early remnant of what we have come to understand as nursing diagnosis, or an appreciation of the patients' perspective regarding their illness. It can also be seen as acknowledging the psychosocial aspects of physical illness. Regardless of the interpretation, the criterion points to the necessity of communicating with patients in order to identify and incorporate their perceptions.

INFLUENCE OF PSYCHIATRIC–MENTAL HEALTH NURSING

It was in the clinical specialty of psychiatric nursing that the concepts and theories of communication and the nurse–patient relationship were to be developed and introduced into the entire discipline of nursing. Most schools of nursing did not offer a separate clinical experience or theory portion focused on psychiatric–mental health until quite late. By 1944 there were still 14 states that had no psychiatric courses in their nursing programs (Kalisch & Kalisch, 2004). The change to having psychiatric nursing included in nursing curricula is credited to the efforts of Effie Taylor. A graduate of Johns Hopkins School of Nursing in 1904, Taylor later studied at Teachers College, Columbia University, and Yale's Department of Public Health. Her career included serving as Associate Principle at Johns Hopkins School of Nursing until 1922, Superintendent of the Connecticut Training School (later named Yale University School of Nursing), and second Dean of Yale's School of Nursing. It was Taylor's interest in *patient-centered* care that led her to arrive at a different model for nursing. Under her leadership, nurses were assigned to specific patients instead of specific tasks, such as dispensing medications or obtaining vital signs for all patients on a floor. Her model was clearly the beginning of what was later referred to as primary nursing. The ability to form a relationship with a patient and family over time, even if during a brief hospitalization, promotes continuity of care. The model also relieves the nurses from being purely task oriented, and places the patient at the center of their work. The patient's emotional and intellectual state was also emphasized in this model of providing care (Church, 1988; Friedman, 1988).

It was Taylor's involvement in professional nursing organizations, however, that allowed her to influence the national scene of nursing curriculum revision. In 1932, Taylor was President of the NLNE and it was during her 4-year term that *A Curriculum Guide for Schools of Nursing* (1937) was being developed. Although this curriculum guide suggested that psychiatric nursing be included in all nursing curricula, the emphasis of the guide was on medical–surgical procedures and skills. The functional nursing model, which originated in the 1930s, was developed by Isabel Stewart and instituted in most hospital schools of nursing in the late 1960s. It stressed procedural expertise without emphasis on the underlying principles, making nursing care rule-based and activity oriented, stressing repetition and neglect of the psychosocial aspects of patient care. Nursing practice in this model was taught without much regard for an intellectual understanding on the part of the clinician of the principles underlying the procedures (Fairman, 2002). In order to address this problem, basic and behavioral sciences were introduced to nursing curricula during the 1950s. Regardless of this shift, according to an NLN report almost a decade later, the integration of basic and behavioral sciences into clinical practice was still problematic (NLN, 1959).

It was clear that a different approach to patient care was needed and an alternative perspective was offered by several nursing pioneers including Hildegard Peplau, Ester Lucille Brown, and Virginia Henderson. Henderson was yet another leader who consistently called for the inclusion of psychiatric nursing into the standard nursing curricula. Henderson reflected on her own early nursing training:

> *Most of my training was in a general hospital where, for the nurse, technical competence, speed of performance, and a "professional" (actually an impersonal) manner were stressed. We were introduced to nursing as a series of almost unrelated procedures, beginning with an unoccupied bed and progressing to aspiration of body cavities, for instance. Ability to catheterize a patient in this era seemed to qualify a student for so-called night duty, where, without any previous experience in the administration of a service, she might have the entire care of as many as 30 sick souls and bodies* (Henderson, 1991, p. 10).

Henderson's career began as a visiting nurse, as was typical during that time, and then progressed to nursing education where she remained at Teachers College, Columbia University, for two decades. It was during this time that she developed and expanded her definition of nursing. She was also influenced by her colleagues at Columbia in the areas of physiology, psychology, and rehabilitation. Henderson brought all of this knowledge and experience to bear as she joined others in the 1937 revision of the NLNE's basic curriculum guide. Henderson tested out her ideas at Columbia during the 1940s in an advanced medical–surgical course that was patient-centered and was organized around nursing situations instead of medical diagnoses. It was a pioneer course, in that students were allowed to provide care under a case assignment system allowing for comprehensive care, including follow-up patient care.

Virginia Henderson was later influenced by Gwen Tudor Will and Ida Orlando Pelletier (*The Dynamic Nurse-Patient Relationship*, 1959) and Ernestine Wiedenback (*Clinical Nursing: A Helping Art*, 1964). She was interested in examining the true nature of nursing and she continued to define the profession, always with an emphasis on the patient. In the presentation of her work, Henderson provided an interesting visual concerning nursing in her depiction of health and medical care in the form a pie graph, assigning wedges of various sizes to members of the healthcare team. She attempted to make the point, whether for the comatose postsurgical patient or the newborn infant, that it was nursing care that played the major role (Henderson, 1991).

Psychiatric nursing leaders emphasized the importance of understanding patient's needs and coined various communication techniques as *validation* and *clarification*. During the 1950s and 1960s, Hildegard Peplau (known as the mother of psychiatric nursing), Brown (a sociologist), and Virginia Henderson were the trio who voiced concern about the discrepancy between what nurses were taught and what patients needed. They called for a focus on individual patient assessment and care. As a result of their efforts, the patients' *affective experience* regarding their physical problems became an important part of what was considered good nursing care. It was coined *interpersonal care* and was supported by research generated from various applied and social sciences (Fawcett, 2005).

Hildegard Peplau and Her Influences

Hildegard Peplau is credited with identifying and exploring the concept of the nurse–patient relationship. Her contribution was highlighting the importance of the relationship, regardless of clinical setting or population. Although she was a psychiatric–mental health nurse, her belief about this relationship extended to all nurses working with all patients in any setting. The nurse–patient theory is a middle-range descriptive classification theory that focuses on phases of the nurse–patient interaction. Peplau believed that only by understanding the interaction from the *patient's* perspective could the nurse be truly effective. She was less interested in pathophysiology or psychopathology as it was the person-to-person human experience that interested her. Peplau was particularly concerned when someone was "ill" and trying to address issues related to health (Peplau, 1952). Interpersonal relationships formed the "core of nursing" regardless of whether the nurse is engaged in a teaching role or carrying out a technical procedure (Peplau, 1964). Peplau's interpersonal theory is equally applicable for advanced practice nurses as for undergraduate or basic students and, considering the skill required, perhaps even more so. Like the late entry of actual psychiatric nursing theory and clinical rotations in nursing education, psychiatric principles were also late arrivals. Schmahl (1966) conducted a 5-year study of this issue at Skidmore and confirmed that true integration of psychiatric principles, even at this late date, although beneficial, was not the accepted norm in nursing education.

In the mid-20th century objectivity was singularly valued in academic settings and positivistic research was the only path to professional credibility. Nursing was working hard to find a seat at the table and the scientific method and model was adopted in order to secure such a seat. It has been argued that this philosophy may have served to cripple the artistic, nonquantifiable elements of nursing care. Understanding the history of how knowledge development in nursing evolved is critical to freeing nurses from the "conceptual ghetto" identified by Clouser in which members of a profession are "locked into a certain way of seeing the world" (AAHN, 2001).

Creative ways of viewing patient care delivery and educational methods of teaching communication skills require that educators honor more than

gs and the results garnered from meta-analyses. Communi-
aboratories are an example of a novel method of teaching
...ucation skills. Simulation has been shown to be an effective adjunct
to didactic instruction. Simulation allows students to practice empathetic communication skills, delivering "bad news," and conduct motivational interviewing, which utilizes open-ended questions (Rosenzweig et al., 2008).

In juxtaposition to an emphasis on procedures and techniques, an exciting new model of care has developed that is primarily concerned with the *patient* as the focus. It has been dubbed patient-centered, and one could ask who else should be at the center, if not the patient? It is also important to place all interventions within the context of the nurse–patient relationship. An interesting and disturbing study of this relationship suggests that educational/occupational status continues to be a source of power for nurses within this relationship and patients may feel powerless when dealing with their provider (Oudshoorn, Ward-Griffin, & McWilliam, 2000). The authors recommend that nurses reflect on and change the disempowering aspects of the nurse–client relationship in order to improve home-based palliative care. Mok and Chiu (2004) studied the nurse–patient relationship in the context of palliative care and found that the presence or absence of a trusting relationship was paramount. In this study nurses became "part of the family" as well as providers of care and, because of the trust from patients and families, they were more capable of providing holistic care, to demonstrate their understanding of patient suffering, and to provide comfort measures in an intuitive manner. Based on trust, the goals of both nurse and patient could be achieved along with demonstrated caring and a sense of reciprocity in the relationship. This quality of relationship has demonstrated positive effects in regard to improvement of both physical and emotional issues, illness adjustment on the part of the patient, and ultimately effective pain management and a positive death experience. In addition, as a result of this approach, the nurse can experience a sense of satisfaction and enrichment as a result of being in a relationship with another human being that has genuine meaning.

PATIENT-CENTERED CARE

Effective patient care requires attending as much to patient's personal experiences of illness as to their diseases (Stewart et al., 1995, p. 27).

The model of patient-centered care is founded on the work of Carl Rodgers, Balint (1957), and Neuman and Young (1972) who adapted the model for nursing. Patient-centered care means embracing the concept of patient and family collaboration. This collaboration can be accomplished in a variety of ways, including actively seeking patient and family participation in decision making and teaching patients self-management skills. Patient-centered approaches emphasize the clinician's style of communication, the use of empathy, and the ability to manage the emotional reactions of patients.

A Commonwealth Fund survey found that most patients, between 30 and 80%, reported that their needs during a primary care visit were not met. This was attributed to less-than-optimal communication between patient and clinician, inadequate time for patients to talk, and exclusion of patients from decision making (Epstein, Mauksch, Carroll, & Jaen, 2008). There is ample evidence that patients desire both more information as well as more involvement in medical decision making (Coulter, 1997).

Research on training healthcare providers in this area reveals that clinician's patient-centeredness results in improved patient communication, clarification of patient concerns, and greater patient satisfaction (Lewin, Entwistle, Zwarenstein, & Dick, 2001). During the medical interview, Barrier and Jensen (2003) refer to the "essential functions" of gathering information, building a relationship, and educating the patient. Merely asking the question "What else?" was found to be linked to an improvement in health outcomes, patient compliance, and patient satisfaction, as well as a reduction in malpractice suits.

The value of a caring relationship with patients continues to be important to advanced practice nurses particularly because of the tension created when productivity concerns dominate a clinical setting, such as in primary care (Green, 2004). Advanced practice nurses are called on to coordinate care between patients and multiple providers as well as teach patients effective resource utilization, including use of the Internet for seeking medical information and in assisting in overall communications with healthcare providers.

Various models of care exist that address the challenges of the time constraint inherent in the primary care setting and yet stay true to the conceptual framework of patient-centered care (Box 1-2).

Focus Protocol

Epstein et al. (2008) propose a series of steps to be followed in primary care in an effort to set an agenda in a collaborative fashion with a patient. The steps involve:

1. Ask about *all* of the patient's concerns
2. Develop a working agenda
3. Sort through the patient's concerns and prioritize
4. Structure the office visit with the previous steps in mind

Box 1-2   Nursing Education Models

Name	Authors	Description
Patient-centered care	Carl Rodgers, Neuman & Young	Collaboration between patient, family, healthcare team
Focus protocol	Epstein et al.	Establish agenda with patient
Three function approach	AACH, Mayo Clinic	Gather information, build relationship, educate patient
Four habits approach	Frankel, Stein, & Krupat	Invest in the beginning, elicit patient perspective, empathize, invest in the end
Family-centered care	Institute for Family-Centered Care	Importance of family as support network and healthcare advisors; core concepts: dignity and respect, information sharing, participation, collaboration
Nurse–patient theory	Hildegard Peplau	Focus on phases of nurse–patient relationship
Patient-centered approach	Univ. of Western Ontario	Six components (see Box 1-3)
Patient-centered care model	Picker Institute	Discover needs and concerns of patients/family to provide better health care
Reflective practice	Donald Schon	Reflection-in-action
Clinical practice development model	Patricia Benner	Seven domains of expert care; beginning of phenomenology

In addition to guiding the office visit, the authors suggest that clinicians communicate with patients before a visit, either utilizing online forms or written materials that ask patients to list their concerns and invite them to participate in the visit by preparing questions ahead of time. This strategy will save time during the actual visit and help both the patient and clinician to accomplish the goals for the visit.

The Three Function Approach

The American Academy on Communication in Healthcare (AACH) has developed institutional workshops for physicians, the "three function" approach for effective physician–patient communication, developed at the Mayo Clinic. They cite the statistic that, according to a Commonwealth Fund survey, more than 30% of respondents reported leaving a doctor's office without getting an answer to an important question. Half reported that the doctor did not discuss the emotional aspects of their illness, including coping skills or strategies.

The three functions are:

1. *Information gathering*: allowing patients to tell their story and using prompts that assure the whole story is elicited, thereby setting an agenda for the clinical visit.
2. *Relationship building*: using PEARLS, or

   Partnership
   Empathy
   Apology
   Respect
   Legitimization
   Support

3. *Patient education*: using "tell and ask," a combination of providing information and then asking about specific patient concerns *before* advancing to another piece of information.

Four Habits Approach

Frankel, Stein, and Krupat (2003) developed four habits of physician–patient communication that has been taught at Kaiser Permanente since 1996. The habits are:

1. *Invest in the beginning*: start with open-ended questions and then prioritize the patient's concerns.
2. *Elicit the patient's perspective*, including their thoughts on etiology as well as concerns and expectations for care.
3. *Demonstrate empathy*.
4. *Invest in the end*: frame the diagnosis in terms of the patient's original concerns and inquire about patient satisfaction.

The original model of patient-centered care is now also referred to as "family-centered" care. The Institute for Family-Centered Care defines this model as an approach to planning, delivering, and evaluating health care that is based on "mutually beneficial partnerships" among patients, families, and providers regardless of setting or specific patient population related to age or clinical condition. The Institute for Family-Centered Care is a nonprofit organization founded in 1992 whose mission is to advance the understanding and practice of patient- and family-centered care. The shift from the patient to the family acknowledges the central place families have in a patient's support network and honors the importance of families as advisors and partners when improving clinical care and systems of delivering that care. The Institute for Family-Centered Care also notes that people most dependent on hospital care and use of the healthcare system are also often most dependent on families. This population includes the very young, the very old, and those with chronic conditions. The Institute identifies the "core concepts" patient- and family-centered care as:

Dignity and Respect
Information Sharing
Participation
Collaboration

These core concepts require active listening on the part of healthcare providers, and a nonjudgmental approach. Information is shared in a timely, complete, and accurate manner in order to allow patients and families to make decisions about health care. Participation is encouraged and supported and patients and families are asked for input in regard to wider institutional, policy, and program issues. Williamson (2005) notes that it is often difficult to distinguish between policies that are withheld because of the clinician's personal or clinical views and those that represent the rationing of services. Because of this, the following suggestions are offered for the provider in order to preserve the clinical relationship and to support the patient's autonomy.

1. Offer easy access to institutional and clinical policies and guidelines that may affect the patient.
2. Make available unwritten policies.
3. Decide how to make available to patients any policies that are unwritten.
4. Consider discussing with patient groups how to offer information about policies that may be distressing to patients.

The patient-centered model is a natural for the profession of nursing, which utilizes a biopsychosocial model, and the foundational element of the nurse–patient relationship. In this model, the provider reaches an understanding of the patient's illness by placing themselves in the patient's shoes, a technique stressed by Carl Rodgers. As clinicians, we cannot assume that we know what meaning the illness holds for a patient or family. It is dangerous to lump patients and families together and to generalize from our past experiences. No matter how expert or seasoned the clinician is, it is critical that the provider does not make assumptions, no matter how similar the patient may be to past patients they have treated. Patients and families are unique, and require a suspension of judgment and a willingness to enter the patient's world. This may be accomplished by being attentive to the patient's ideas, expectations, feelings, and conducting discussions regarding the effect of illness on their ability to function on a day-to-day basis. It demands that the provider set aside an image of what *they* would be feeling or thinking if they experienced a particular diagnosis or treatment option. This strategy requires the clinician to identify the subtle and not so subtle cues that the patient or family provides during a clinical encounter. Utilizing the patient-centered approach in the clinical setting might lead to a variety of questions, including:

What is the patient's understanding of the illness?
What does the patient believe caused it?
What are his or her expectations of the provider?
What are his or her feelings?
What are his or her fears?

Toombs (1992) has stated that all patients want to be understood, appreciated, and recognized. In order to meet these needs, clinicians must avoid attending to only the superficial words that patients present and must be willing to dig deeper. Instead of quickly categorizing patients according to specific diagnostic criteria, providers must understand the person at a deeper level. This model requires that the clinician place the initial symptoms in a very *personal* context and avoid making judgments and assumptions. It requires the ability and the willingness to truly listen. Stewart et al. (1995) refers to this process as "responding to suffering." This process requires a departure from responding only to physical complaints and concerns. It demands seeing the patient as a complex person, who lives within a complex system that is dynamic, and as someone capable of affecting one's own health status. It assumes that the patient arrives to the consultation with a set of ideas concerning their illness. A patient's symptoms have meaning for them and this will probably only be revealed *if* the clinician directly inquires about this *meaning*. Therefore, specific questions need to be posed to patients and families that elicit this information. Patients and families also experience understandable fears about symptoms or illness. This is another area that may remain underground and unexplored if not directly asked by the clinician. It is important not to assume you know what a patient is feeling about *any* aspect of their health or illness. "Tell me about your feelings" is much preferred to "You must be feeling anxious." The clinician may have an intuitive feeling about what the patient or family is feeling, but it is more effective to not lead the conversation in any specific direction. Patients and families that are trying to please or who are easily influenced will sometimes agree with a leading statement rather than contradict a clinician. The theory and practice of "active listening" will be further explored in Chapter 4.

Patient-Centered Approach

A specific patient-centered approach, contrasted to the medical-centered approach, has been developed at the University of Western Ontario (Levenstein, McCracken, McWhinney, Stewart, & Brown, 1986). The model consists of six components, see Box 1-3.

This model is particularly well suited in the setting of primary care and, specifically, family practice. It incorporates the clinician's exploration of both the patient's disease and dimensions of the illness experience, including feelings about being ill, a patient's ideas about what ails them, the impact of the problem on their daily functioning, and their expectations of what should be done. This model also emphasizes a holistic approach and, therefore, is particularly well

---

Box 1-3   Six Components of University of Western Ontario's Patient-Centered Care Model

Explore both the disease and the illness experience: differential diagnoses; dimensions of illness, including feelings and expectations	Prevention and health promotion: health enhancement, risk reduction, early disease detection, ameliorating effects of disease
Understand the whole person: the person includes life story, personal and developmental issues; the context includes family or anyone else affected by the patient's illness	Enhance the relationship: characteristics of a therapeutic relationship, sharing power, caring and healing relationship, self-awareness, transference and countertransference
Find common ground in regard to management: problems and priorities, treatment goals, clarification of roles of provider and patient	Realism: time, resources, team building

Stewart et al., 1995, p. 25

suited from a nursing perspective. An additional component of the model is the search for establishing common ground with a patient or family in regard to the management of health and illness, thus incorporating health promotion and prevention. Also central to the model is an emphasis on the patient–provider relationship and a requirement that the practice be realistic.

Studies that have focused on the benefits of the patient-centered model have reported better patient satisfaction (Roter, 1989), better provider satisfaction (Roter et al., 1997), fewer malpractice complaints (Levinson, Roter, Mullooly, Dull, & Frankel, 1997), and, contrary to popular belief, the approach does *not* increase the time of a typical office visit (Roter et al., 1997). Although this model was developed to address what the authors considered a troubled physician–patient relationship, it is a useful model for advanced practice nurses and graduate level healthcare providers.

Question Builder

The Agency for Healthcare Research and Quality (AHRQ), part of the US Department of Health and Human Services, has developed a tool for assisting patients in preparing for a visit to a healthcare provider. This tool is referred to as Question Builder, and it aims to help the patient clarify the purpose of the visit, by asking:

Did your clinician give you a prescription?
Are you scheduled to have medical tests?
Did you recently receive a diagnosis?
Are you considering treatment for an illness or condition?
Did your clinician recently recommend surgery?
Are you choosing a health plan?
Are you choosing a clinician?
Are you choosing a hospital?
Are you choosing long-term care?

After choosing a category, the patient is guided through a series of relevant questions that are useful to address during a clinical visit. For example, for patients considering treatment for an illness or condition, the questions are:

What are my treatment options?
What do you recommend?
Is the treatment painful?
How can the pain be controlled?
What are the benefits and risks of this treatment?

How much does this treatment cost?
Will my health insurance cover the treatment?
What are the expected results?
When will I see results from the treatment?
What are the chances the treatment will work?
Are there any side effects?
What can be done about them?
How soon do I need to make a decision about treatment?
What happens if I choose to have no treatment at all?

Lang, Floyd, and Beine (2000) explore the presence of clues that patients present during a routine office visit that are often missed. These clues relate to how patients perceive their illness and arrive in a variety of forms, including:

Direct statements about the impact of an illness
Expressions of feelings about the illness, including nonverbal expressions
Attempts to explain symptoms, without naming an illness
Repetition of ideas about an illness
Asking loaded questions
The presence of another person during the visit
Interruptions of the clinician by the patient
Scheduling a routine visit without a specific presenting complaint
Resisting a recommendation
Expressing dissatisfaction with previous care
Sharing a personal story during a visit

Utilizing a patient-centered approach begins with the first utterance by the clinician, "What brings you to the clinic today?" and the follow-up response to the patient's answer to the question. The clinician will choose to only focus on the symptoms that are reported or will venture into the world of ideas, feelings, and functional aspects that are related to the presenting complaints. How often in the traditional medical model is the patient asked about what *their* thoughts about the symptoms or illness are? Michael Crichton, better known for his thriller novels rather than his medical skills, wrote about his dissatisfaction with the traditional medical approach during his clinical rotations at Beth Israel Hospital during his final year at Harvard Medical School in the 1960s (Crichton, 1988). He decided, during his rotation on the cardiac unit, to ask patients who had experienced a heart attack what ideas they had about *why* they had suffered a cardiac event. He reports that patients quickly responded to the question with various theories, and Crichton marveled at the fact that this question was not part of the interview process he was taught to conduct. The patients were typically middle-aged men who had various thoughts about the meaning of their illnesses when asked "Why did you have a heart attack?" Although the young medical student worried that the question might anger some patients because it implied a sense of control, he found that instead of anger, patients would validate that they had been thinking about just that question. The stories that patients told were of various events that had literally broken their hearts. They were stories of lost love, rejection, and events in which their hearts had been "attacked." It led the young medical student to the conclusion that the relationship between mind, heart, and illness was underappreciated in his medical education. Although Michael Crichton left medicine, once his book *Andromeda Strain* was sold to be made into a movie, his experiences speak to the notion of understanding the meaning of a symptom or illness for the patient. Levenstein, McCracken, McWhinney, Stewart, and Brown (1986) make a clear distinction between *disease* and *illness* when developing the foundations of the patient-centered model. The disease is what we try to categorize and find a code for reimbursement purposes. It is helpful in terms of communicating with other healthcare professionals to use this frame. This view may drive treatment choices and tell us something about prognosis and recovery. It may say something about etiology and inform us in regard to what is to be expected in future. However, it is not in any way individual or personal. It does not take into account the many variables that we know play a part in how the course of treatment will proceed. In addition, this view helps clinicians distance themselves from patients. Some may prefer it as a method because it is generalized and perhaps even cut and dry. It is not plagued by the messiness of all of the unique variables that the concept of illness brings to mind. Whereas a disease is a concept of something outside of the person, an illness is a lived experience that is very much a part of the person. No two will be the same, and the onus is on the healthcare provider to attempt to uncover the nuances that make the patient's perspective clear. A natural curiosity and humility is required with this approach, and it directly competes with the authoritative expert posture of the clinician who, once pouncing on a diagnosis, has all of the information and answers. Although pathophysiology is important, it is simply not enough. It places the emphasis on cells and physiology, not on the person. Mishler (1984) refers to turning away from a scientific, detached posture to one that pays attention to the social context, the meaning of an illness event, and the subsequent affect on personal goals as a "lifeworld" approach. Asking a patient what most concerns them, how it is disruptive to their life, and how they think you can be helpful is useful when following this approach.

In writing about the various stages of illness, Reiser and Schroder (1980) identified three stages: awareness, disorganization, and reorganization. This is similar to human response to trauma or a disaster. It would seem logical that a clinician needs to place any communication in the context of this process. For example, to give copious direction initially, when the patient is struggling with new information, seems foolish. Initially, patients would expect to be in some form of denial, an expected defense mechanism that is unconscious. Patients will typically be highly ambivalent about knowing too much, while wanting the truth at the same time. Another struggle involves a wish to be cared for and a desire to maintain independence. If symptoms persist, issues of a diminished sense of control are predictable. In disorganization, patients regress and may relate to their provider as a parental figure. They may be cranky, demanding, and irritable. Others may become withdrawn, sullen, and lose hope. This difficult stage requires sensitivity on the part of the clinician if they hope to be effective. Finally, in the third stage, a patient seeks a new understanding in the face of illness. Social support plays an important role as does the relationship with the healthcare provider.

Challenges to patient-centered care (Holmes, Cramer, & Charns, 2003) include the fact that a certain treatment requested by a patient or family may not be supported by evidence-based practice. Some clinicians may not be comfortable with patients and families who are fully engaged with their care, preferring a more traditional passive patient role. Not all patients or families will be confident in their right to be involved in treatment decisions or have confidence in their opinions, leading to discomfort in regard to fully participating with healthcare providers. In addition, healthcare providers may be leery for patients and families to know too much, fearing litigation.

THE PICKER INSTITUTE

"Understanding and respecting patient's values, preferences and expressed needs is the foundation of patient-centered care."

—Harvey Picker

A patient-centered care model was also developed in 1984 at the Picker Institute, by Harvey and Jean Picker, as a result of their personal experience with the healthcare system. The Institute has the goal of improving healthcare delivery from the perspective of paying attention to patient's needs and listening to the concerns of patients and family members. This not-for-profit organization led the movement to develop a scholarly approach to discovering the needs and concerns of patients and families in order to assist healthcare professionals. Researchers developed new performance measurement tools after finding that the tools available at the time, aimed at measuring patient satisfaction, did not truly measure patient preference. The Picker Institute believes that patients' views and experiences are "integral" to the effort to improve patient care. The principles that guide this patient-centered approach include:

Physical comfort and a safe environment
Empathy and emotional support
Involvement of family and friends
Fast access to reliable health advice
Effective treatment delivered by trustworthy staff
Continuity of care
Involvement in decisions and respect for patient preferences

The original survey utilized at the Institute was aimed at answering the following questions:

What do patients want?
What do patients value?
What helps or hinders their ability to manage health problems?
What aspects of care are most important to patients and families?

The Institute has further refined the survey in order to address the results of the original Picker survey and addresses the following areas:

Access: including time spent waiting for admission or time between admission and allocation to a bed in a ward

Respect for patient's values, preferences, and expressed needs: including the impact of illness and treatment on quality of life, involvement in decision making, dignity, needs, and autonomy

Coordination and integration of care: including clinical care, ancillary and support services, and "front-line" care

Information, communication, and education: including clinical status, progress and prognosis, facilitation of autonomy, self-care, and health promotion

Physical comfort: including pain management, help with activities of daily living, surroundings, and hospital environment

Emotional support and alleviation of fear and anxiety: including treatment and prognosis, impact of illness on self and family, financial impact of illness

Involvement of family and friends: including social and emotional support, involvement in decision making, impact on family dynamics and functioning

Transition and continuity: including information about medication and danger signs to look out for after leaving the hospital, coordination and discharge planning, and clinical, social, physical, and financial support

The Picker survey is analyzed by the creation of 40 "problem scores," which indicate the presence or absence of problems. These are then summarized into "dimension scores" according to theme. More than 8000 patients, family members, and healthcare providers were involved in the original research. In addition to uncovering invaluable information about what areas of care most mattered to patients and families, the survey used a new approach: that of asking patients and families to report on their experience of health care instead of the typical patient satisfaction rating survey. Now this method of measuring performance, from the perspective of the patient and family, is considered a standard. Today the Picker Institute surveys are utilized not only in the United States, but also in Great Britain, Sweden, Germany, and Switzerland. The surveys provide patient experience measurement services to the healthcare industry and sponsors education and research in the area of patient-centered care.

An example of information derived from the Picker survey is a study about the harmful effects and ethical and political implications of withholding information from patients about organizational policies (Williamson, 2005). This practice of withholding information can undermine patient autonomy and repress their political voice. These results underscore the connection between offering patients and families access to policies and ethical clinical practice.

REFLECTIVE PRACTICE

When nurses welcome patient's feelings, respect their wishes, and honor their need for self-expression, they help patient's choose options that are in their best interest (Appleton, 1994, p.103).

It was an educator, Donald Schön (1987), who first introduced the concept of reflective practice as a process that taught teachers how to hone their skills. Schön's work grew out of what he called a "crisis of confidence" in teaching when there existed the pressure for a better educated populace in the face of increasing competition and Asian imports. He was interested in "reflection-in-action" or what teachers did in classrooms. Reflection-in-action is a response based on improvisation, and it is artistic. It often is initiated when the practitioner is surprised, and then puzzled, and then responds with an on-the-spot experiment based on an understanding of what is occurring. It requires thought about the surprise and an awareness of looking at or reflecting while doing. It leads to new ways of behaving if the experiment brings a positive result. The practitioner can then store the experience for future use in similar situations. Schön called it "thought turning back on itself." He likened it to jazz and good conversation, where neither is wholly predictable. Schön also confessed that teaching students to do something he did well was indeed challenging unless he reflected on *how* he did the thing, or observed himself at least mentally. He warned that theories only take one so far when trying to teach.

Schön encouraged both the novice as well as the seasoned professional to actively engage in a process of reflecting on one's experiences and then applying the knowledge to future encounters. He argued that reflection-on-action was intellectual work requiring verbalization. He eloquently spoke of the separation of research and practice in the modern university that has little tolerance for artistry, messiness, and nontechnical problem solving. "The challenge to the professional schools, I think, is this challenge of educating for artistry. Helping people become more competent in the indeterminate zones of practice, as carrying out processes of reflection-on-action and reflection ON reflection-in-action" (Schön, 1987). Schön called on various professional schools to pick up the gauntlet, including athletics, arts, architecture, music, and dance and nursing. He believed in a "reflective practicum" whose main feature is a situation in which people learn by *doing*; with others involved in the same activity in a virtual world, students can run experiments cheaply and without great danger. "They don't have to actually go out and build a building to learn about designing a building. And they don't have to go out and kill a patient to learn what the carotid artery is. And they can actually go back and do it again, and they can control the pace of the doing. I believe, the experience of students in any reflective practicum is that they must plunge into the doing, and try to educate themselves before they know what it is they're trying to learn. *The teachers cannot tell them*" (Schön, 1987, p. 12).

Initially implemented in colleges of education, reflective practice is a natural fit for many healthcare disciplines. Like Benner's continuum model, Schön's model is based on different levels of practice. The popular portfolio utilized for both admission and graduation requirements in many fields are an example of the homage paid to the theory of reflective practice.

Reflective Practice and Nursing

Awareness of personal and professional values enhances clinical judgment for the advanced practice nurse (Chase, 2004). These values include openness, courage, persistence, and loyalty to patients. Reflection is the path to understanding one's beliefs and values. Although educators struggle to find ways to incorporate reflective writing in the curriculum, once accomplished, student writing improves over time (Epp, 2008).

Although there are several models for reflective practice in nursing, Johns (2007) defines and describes reflection as:

> *Reflection is being mindful of self, either within or after experience, as if a window through which the practitioner can view and focus self within the context of a particular experience, in order to confront, understand and move toward resolving contradiction between one's vision and actual practice. Though the conflict of contradiction, the commitment to realize one's vision, and understanding why things are as they are, the practitioner can gain new insights into self and be empowered to respond more congruently in future situations within a reflexive spiral towards developing practical wisdom and realizing one's vision as a lived reality. The practitioner may require guidance to overcome resistance or to be empowered to act on understanding (p. 2).*

In other words, reflection involves intuition, perception, and cognition based on a lived experience with a patient in order to understand ourselves and how we may practice more effectively. Johns has outlined a model that incorporates various ways of knowing. It calls for the practitioner to first recall the interaction in one's mind and then focus on one part of the experience that seemed to be significant. Then the practitioner focuses on what others were feeling and why, and then how they were feeling and why. Next, the clinician thinks about what exactly they were trying to achieve in the interaction and how effective they were. The clinician asks what the consequences were for the patient, others involved, and for them. Following this, the practitioner looks inward and asks what factors influenced how they felt, thought, and behaved. What knowledge informed or might have informed? They then assess how the behavior matches up with their value system, prior similar experiences, and how they might be more effective in future. Alternative actions are considered in terms of consequences for the patient, others, and self. Finally, the practitioner assesses how they now feel having gone through the prior set of questions (Johns, 2005).

Role play and reverse role play are methods used to facilitate the process of reflection by simulating Socratic dialogue (Todd, 2005). Students can either be in diads or a triad. In the latter configuration, students take the role of patient or nurse, and the third person's role is to observe, offer technical prompts, and help guide the interaction.

Homework assignments are an integral part of reflection. This can be in the form of a reflective journal which records clinical practice situations that line up with classroom activities and theory. In a reflective journal thoughts and affect can be explored alongside behavior in order to lead to increased self-awareness and be used as a guide for future practice. A reflective journal assists clinicians in identifying specific learning experiences as well as recording professional growth as the clinician moves from novice to expert. Jasper (2003) has clarified that the connection between reflective writing and learning occurs because writing helps to:

Order our thinking
Develop analytical skills
Develop critical thinking skills
Develop creativity
Identify and clarify the limits of understanding

In addition to these, Moon (1999) has identified the purposes of keeping a journal:

Encourage metacognititon
Enhance problem-solving skills
Serve as a form of self-expression
Increase participation in one's own learning
Enhance personal development
Enhance self-empowerment
Foster communication and interaction in a group
Support planning and progress in scholarly projects

Kim (1999) has developed a method of inquiry meant to assist clinicians in being critical thinkers who are reflective in regard to their practice. The phases of this inquiry include a descriptive phase, a reflective phase, and a critical phase. Practitioners develop descriptive narratives that are used to promote self-awareness and new knowledge as a result of reflection. Finally, a critique of practice leads to new learning and a change in practice. The goal is to learn to identify good versus ineffective practice, to generate knowledge from practice, and to change or correct ongoing practice. There is value to allowing students to utilize reflective writing with some distance from the actual clinical encounter, including both actual patients and the clinical site. In one model, Web journaling provides the opportunity for faculty and students to dialogue about clinical situations, and can raise the awareness of both students and faculty in regard to the learning needs of the students and their evolving understanding of their patients (Cohen & Welch, 2002). Because this method is Web-based, students are encouraged to utilize the Internet for information. Faculty guide students in the use of the information, with particular patients under specific circumstances. Use of this model over several courses may reinforce the value of both reflective journaling as well as self-directed learning.

> *Web journaling* is a practice that incorporates the principles of journaling, reflective practice, and encouraging students to be self-directed.

THE WORK OF PATRICIA BENNER

A complex social practice such as nursing requires attentive caring relationships with patients and families, professional commitment to develop practical knowledge, astute clinical judgments across time about particular patients and families, and good collaborative relationships with others on the health care team (Benner in Haag-Heitman, 1999, p. 17).

Patricia Benner's work on the attributes of expert practice has served to guide all advanced practice (nurse practitioners, clinical specialists, nurse-midwives, and nurse anesthetists) to common ground in regard to what constitutes advanced practice. In describing "expert," Benner identified seven domains: the helping role; the teaching–coaching function; effective management of rapidly changing situations; diagnostic and patient monitoring role; monitoring interventions and regimens; ensuring quality in healthcare practices; and organizational competencies. It was Fenton (1983) who applied these domains in order to further clarify advanced or graduate nursing practice. Brykcyznski (1989) studied nurse practitioners in outpatient care settings and added a domain related to ambulatory care. Studies focusing on advanced practice nurses' communications styles, which enable health promotion and disease prevention, are in the early stages (Berry, 2006).

In discussing clinical decision making for the advanced practice nurse, Smith (2006) suggests the following approaches:

Understand the meaning that patients attribute to their health.

Learn about the patient's lived social world, support system, and role responsibilities.

Along with the patient, note personal and social health obstacles and facilitators.

Determine the patient's preference for and ability to participate in health-care decision making and health management.

Mutually set health goals and priorities.

Identify and treat patients in crisis, transitions, and times of loss.

Know the patient's spiritual framework.

These previously listed approaches require the development and building of a relationship with patients, and this can only be accomplished through effective therapeutic communication.

The art of nursing is the art/act of the experience-in-the-moment. It is the direct apprehension of a situation, the intuitive and embodied knowing that arises from the practice/praxis of nursing. Art arises from the immediate embodied

*grasp of the situation, the tools or instruments with which the artist works, and
the intuitive knowing of what is to be created in the act* (Chinn, 1994, p. 24).

Benner believed that in order to study caring, the personal and cultural meaning must be examined. Her work provides grounding for the method of phenomenology. She cautioned that because the work of nursing was "contextual," "temporal," and "relational" that the usual task analyses of the work would not be sufficient or accurate. She spoke of *experiential learning* and *practical wisdom* as a more appropriate guide for nursing practice. By using a developmental and interpretative approach, nursing becomes "visible" both to the nurse, who has reflected on their practice, and to the larger organizations, which can validate the work. Benner's methodology of studying novice to expert was observational and narrative in nature. In her role as educator, Benner requires first-person experience narratives of her students. These clinical narratives, a form of reflective practice, are meant to encourage learning about new practice or even clinical errors (Benner in Haag-Heitman, 1999).

In the final stage of Benner's clinical practice development model, the expert practitioner is guided by intuition and a skill derived from and grounded in experience. Their practice can be described as "flexible," "innovative," with a "confident self-directed" approach to clients (Haag-Heitman, 1999). The expert is able to identify their own personal values and place them in context, thereby not interfering with the patient or family and their decisions regarding care. Caring is characterized by being fully present with the patient, "being with" as opposed to "doing to." It requires active listening, understanding the meaning for the patient and family of the current situation. Care also means providing hope offered in the context of a trusting relationship. Only within such a relationship can the provider act as patient advocate, assist in making choices, and truly empower patients and their families.

Clinical intuition or forethought is the ability to make sense of the clinical situation by recognizing patterns and similarities. It means anticipating difficulty and early intervention and an ability to prioritize. Delegation and decisive action are components of this skill, and it requires clear and convincing communication skills in order to explain to colleagues the basis of opinions (Haag-Heitman, 1999).

We stand on the threshold of developing knowledge of the art of nursing and aesthetic knowing in nursing. Breaking new ground is difficult because the ways we have learned to think, to practice, to be, stifle creativity and devalue ways of knowing closely associated with women. As nurses engaged in the process of developing experiential criticism have reflected time and again, moving to new awareness of nursing practice as an art opens remarkable possibilities for the future (Chinn, 1994, p. 37–38).

IMPLICATIONS FOR ADVANCED PRACTICE NURSING

Essential to high-quality clinical judgment is the ability of the nurse practitioner to form a link between patient's life experiences, their problems, and the full range of diagnostic and therapeutic choices available to achieve a range of possible outcomes. The nurse practitioner must be expert at eliciting the true patient story and in recognizing patterns presented in the data (Chase, 2004, p.15).

Jensen (2006) urges advanced practice nurses to honor a different model of patient care, one that acknowledges the contributions of nursing rather than simply adopting the medical model. She stresses that it is not the activities themselves, but rather *how they are carried out* that will differentiate advanced practice nursing from physicians.

The most recent definition of nursing involves protection, promotion, and optimizations of health, prevention of illness, and alleviation of suffering. This is to be accomplished via the processes of diagnosis and treatment and advocacy (ANA, 2003). It is hard to imagine how any of these goals can be accomplished without solid communication skills.

Advanced practice nursing includes clinical specialists, nurse practitioners, nurse anesthetists, and nurse-midwives, and is defined by the ANA scope and standards of practice (2003) as a preparation for specialization, advancement, and expansion of practice. Four common functions of these diverse groups include patient care, educator, researcher, and consultant (Hameric, Spross, & Hanson, 2004). Again, all of these roles require communication skills and one could argue that the complexity of the healthcare system, as well as the expanded scope of practice, require advanced communication knowledge and skills. Advanced practice nurses are leaders in organizations and mentors to other healthcare professionals. There also exists real tension regarding who are the legitimate leaders of a healthcare team that will continue to evolve within the context of an aging population and a nursing shortage. Yet, whether in the clinical arena with families or involved in organization consulting, the advanced practice nurse will need to be a facile and skilled communicator.

The National Association of Clinical Nurse Specialists (NACNS) has described the spheres of influence of the clinical specialist as patients/clients, nurses, and organizations and systems (NACNS, 2004). These spheres of influence form the foundation for the development of core competencies for this group of advanced practice nurses. Communication skills clearly form the basis of functioning in all three spheres.

As the international supply of physicians continues to fail to keep up with demand, and the shifting tide of patient care away from hospitals and into the community advances, the role of advanced practice nurses is increasingly seen as an answer to the question of who will provide care, particularly in the primary care setting. In an attempt to study "nurse–physician substitution" in primary care, a meta-analysis ranging from 1966 to 2002 was done. In all, over 4000 articles were screened and 25 articles were chosen as best relating to inclusion criteria. The analysis found that "no appreciable differences" were discovered between doctors and nurses in regard to health outcomes, actual care, and resource utilization and cost (Laurant, Hermens, Braspenning, Grol, & Sibbald, 2004). In five studies nurses were responsible for initial contact care for patients needing "urgent consultation." In these studies, nurses not only provided longer consultations and more information to patients, but had a higher patient satisfaction grade. In four studies the nurses worked with patients with chronic illnesses and no significant differences were found between doctors and nurses in regard to patient care or financial considerations. The authors concluded that advanced practice nurses can indeed be called on to provide high-quality patient care across the spectrum.

Early studies called the difference between nurse practitioners and physicians "indistinguishable" (Sox, 1979; Stewart et al., 1995), and recent research supports the fact that patients report greater satisfaction regarding care when treated by nurse practitioners. In addition, findings suggest that patients also report receiving longer visits and significantly more information about their illnesses (Hooker, Potts, & Ray, 1997; Kinnersley et al., 2000; Venning, Durie, Roland, Roberts, & Leese, 2000; Horrocks, Anderson, & Salisbury, 2002). In one study, nurse practitioners spent twice as long with their patients and both patients and clinicians spoke more (Seale, Anderson, & Kinnersley, 2005). In addition the nurses talked "significantly more" than general practitioners about treatments and how to apply or carry out treatments. There was also evidence that the nurse practitioners were more likely to discuss social and emotional aspects of patients' lives, discuss the likely course of the patient's condition and side effects of treatments, and use humor.

A recent article in an online journal addressed the issue of communication for nurse practitioners (Katz-Wliner & Feinstein-Whittaker, 2008). The authors, a corporate communication trainer and a speech-language pathologist, offer the following "tips" for effective communication in a clinical encounter:

1. Pay attention to identifying yourself when entering the room, make eye contact, and introduce yourself by name and title.
2. Listen to your patients, attending to both verbal and nonverbal communication without interruption.
3. Avoid using medical jargon and ask patients to repeat all instructions or information in order to assure their understanding of what you are trying to communicate.

4. Speak slowly and clearly.
5. Provide written instructions in regard to any treatment as well as information regarding future appointments and additional resources.
6. Be respectful at all times.
7. Speak directly to the patient, not to family members about the patient, no matter what age the patient.
8. Be professional at all times.
9. Adhere to confidentiality.
10. Be culturally sensitive in your care.

While these authors mention the lessening of "risk exposure," decreased attrition, and decreased patient dissatisfaction as advantages with this approach, they also stress the overall goals of improved patient care and increased image of the clinical practice as well.

COMMUNICATION EXERCISES

1. Patient-Family-Centered Approach

Pair off as patient and provider: 30 minutes.

Provider:

Conduct an initial assessment utilizing four concepts related to the patient-family-centered approach.

Patient:

At the end of the interview try to identify which concepts your provider stressed in the course of the interview.

Discussion:

How does a focus on patient-centered care differ from other assessments you have conducted?

What experiences, as a patient at the receiving end of this approach, were of value?

Were any difficulties encountered, either as patient or provider?

What are the obstacles for implementing this approach in a clinical area?

What changes might you consider for another interview with this approach?

Switch roles and repeat.

2. Patient Understanding of Their Illness

Pair off as patient and provider: 30 minutes.

Provider:

In the process of your interaction with this patient you need to explain a complicated diagnosis, treatment regime, and prognosis.

Patient:

You have just been told of a difficult and complicated diagnosis. You have many questions about treatment as well as fear about your life expectancy. You have a high school diploma and struggled with a learning disorder since grade school. Attempt to communicate your concerns with your clinician as you seek information about your illness.

Discussion:

Debrief the interaction from both the position of the provider and the patient. Explore both the process and the content of the interview, noting any areas when the dialogue became challenging. Share with one another the perspective of patient and provider, while trying to focus on helping a patient understand their illness.

Switch roles and repeat.

_____

_____

_____

_____

_____

_____

_____

_____

_____

_____

_____

_____

_____

_____

_____

_____

3. Patient Expectations

Pair off as patient and provider: 30 minutes.

Provider:

Prepare an initial opening that elicits what the patient is expecting from today's visit.

Patient:

This is the first time seeing this clinician, and you are somewhat reticent. When responding to the question of what you are expecting from the visit, be indirect and somewhat passive. Do not give elaborately detailed responses. Make your provider use their communication skills to draw you out. As the interview unfolds, and you become more comfortable with your provider, you begin to be more open with him/her.

Discussion:

Debrief this interaction from the perspective of how well the patient's expectations were elicited and then addressed.
What were the challenges and successes?
Identify communication techniques that were most useful in this exercise.
Switch roles and repeat.

_____

_____

_____

_____

_____

_____

_____

_____

4. Patient Fears

Pair off as patient and provider: 30 minutes.

Provider:

You are seeing a patient for an annual exam; there are no presenting complaints that you are aware of.

Patient:

You have come to your annual visit with your provider with a serious concern that is particularly embarrassing to you. You are hoping that you will not have to directly express this issue, but that your clinician will ask you about it.

Discussion:

Explore how successful the provider was at uncovering the patient's concerns. What communication techniques were utilized in order to clarify the issues and then deal with the patient's emotional state?
What were the challenges of this exercise?
What learning or insight did you derive from this exercise?
Switch roles and repeat.

_____

_____

_____

_____

_____

_____

_____

_____

5. Patients and Etiology

Pair off as patient and provider: 30 minutes

Provider:

You are seeing a patient who presents with what you have diagnosed as poison ivy. You quickly come to realize that your patient sees this very differently. Use your communication skills to delve into this issue.

Patient:

You have searched the Internet regarding a rash you have developed. You have read both medical sites and blogs discussing rashes and have come to think you have a rare condition that, according to what you have read, is often missed by primary care providers. You are hopeful your provider will listen to your hypothesis.

Discussion:

Debrief this interaction, from the position of patient and provider.
What were the points of tension and how were they dealt with?

Share with one another what it was like to try and communicate your position.

What insight was gained from the exercise? How might you use this understanding in a clinical setting?

Switch roles and repeat.

_____

_____

_____

_____

_____

_____

_____

_____

6. Novice to Expert

Pair off as two providers.

Take turns sharing with one another and identify which stage of professional development you have reached.

Discuss where on the continuum you have reached as a staff nurse and as an advanced practice nurse.

Explore the experience of moving from the role of staff nurse to that of an advanced practice nurse.

What have been the challenges?

What have been the positive aspects of this transition?

_____

_____

_____

_____

_____

_____

_____

_____

7. Nurse–Patient Relationships

Pair off as two providers.

Take turns identifying your personal qualities that facilitate the nurse–patient relationship.

Which qualities do you find most challenging when caring for patients?

Share an experience that best illustrates your ability to engage in a therapeutic relationship with a patient or family.

_____

_____

_____

_____

_____

_____

_____

_____

8. Reflective Practice

Pair off as two providers.

Review the process of reflective practice using a recent clinical event with one another.

Discuss the value of reflective practice in this scenario.

Explore what insights you gained as a result of engaging in reflective thinking about the clinical encounter.

_____

_____

_____

_____

_____

_____

_____

JOURNALING EXERCISES

The unreflective life is not worth living.

—Socrates

Journals have begun to be assigned to students as a method of facilitating reflective practice. Reflection-in-action, as described by Schön (1987), is considered by many to be the cornerstone process of journaling. They are a useful tool for both students and faculty alike for delving more deeply into focused topics. Journaling and role playing, utilized together, can be powerful reinforcers of new learning and promoting critical thinking (Andrusyszyn & Davie, 1997; Halva-Neubauer, 1995). Journaling allows one to bring to conscious awareness new insights and knowledge. The act of reflecting on one's practice cannot help but influence interactions with future patients. Reflective journaling is not simply a matter of recording the events of a day. It requires that the writer identify and examine the underbelly of an experience. What was unclear or confusing? What further questions were generated as a result of the experience? What additional information is needed in order to clarify a confusing aspect of the issue? In these series of journal entries, students will be encouraged to look within in order to increase their self awareness as effective and therapeutic communicators. They will be encouraged to bridge theory and practice with their own personal attributes. Some of the exercises will cause discomfort, but growth rarely occurs where there is no stirring of uneasiness. The value of journaling stems from the fact that it can illuminate contradictions as well as misconceptions. Educational research suggests that active reflection is needed if true transformational learning is to occur. Benefits of journals include clarifying the connections between new knowledge and previous knowledge; examining relationships between what is being learned and the outside world; reflecting on personal goals; sorting out experiences; solving problems; enhancing reflective thinking; enhancing metacognition; improving problem solving and critical thinking; facilitating self-exploration, personal growth, and values clarification; and synthesizing ideas, experiences, and opinions after didactic instruction (Hiemstra, 2001; King & LaRocco, 2006).

1. Nursing History

Discuss your present level of knowledge in regard to nursing history.

What is the relevance of nursing's journey to current practice?

Identify an historical issue that seems to be resurfacing in health care today. What were the lessons of history that can inform today's leaders?

Identify an historical issue that is longstanding and has not reached resolution in nursing.

What are the implications of these historical issues in the current healthcare environment?

Research one of these issues further and prepare to present it in class.

_____

_____

_____

_____

_____

_____

_____

_____

2. The Nurse–Patient Relationship

Discuss what aspects of the relationship you feel most prepared for at this stage of your career.

Your ability to be successful in personal relationships is correlated with your ability to form meaningful nurse–patient relationships. Agree or disagree? Why?

What are the messages you have received in your training regarding patient relationships?

Have you witnessed the nurse–patient relationship as a priority in the clinical settings you have worked?

What interferes with the nurse–patient relationship in your opinion?

What steps can you take to improve in this area?

_____

_____

_____

_____

_____

_____

_____

_____

3. Patient-Centered Care

Discuss your familiarity with this approach before you read this text.

What do you think of the practicality of this approach?

Discuss the challenges of implementing this approach.

What has been your experience with collaborating with patients and families?

Explore the idea that providers lose some power or control when they work in a more collaborative fashion with patients and families.

_____

_____

_____

_____

_____

_____

_____

4. Novice to Expert

Discuss where you see yourself on Benner's continuum of novice to expert.

What implications does Benner's work have for your clinical practice? Be specific.

As you approach the role of an advanced practice nurse, what are the aspects of the role that relate to Benner's theory?

If you are a seasoned clinician returned to graduate studies, how do you see yourself relating to the Benner model?

Do your years of experience mean that you are not a novice as an advanced practice nurse?

Discuss what issues this raises for you.

Does Benner's model match your observations of peers or colleagues?

_____

_____

_____

_____

_____

_____

_____

_____

5. Reflective Practice

Do you consider yourself an introspection person by nature?

What are the challenges of attending to clinical interactions in a thoughtful and reflective manner for you?

What is your experience with keeping a journal?

What do you see as the advantages and drawbacks of keeping a journal of your clinical encounters?

Write about a clinical encounter that you found yourself mentally reviewing long afterward.

Describe the process of "rethinking" how you behaved and responded in this scenario.

What are the implications for future clinical encounters derived from this experience?

Develop and identify goals for yourself as a reflective practitioner.

_____

_____

_____

_____

_____

_____

_____

_____

REFERENCES

American Association for the History of Nurses. (2001). *Nursing history in the curriculum: Preparing nurses for the 21st century.* Wheat Ridge, CO: AAHN.

American Nurses Association. (2003). *Nursing's social policy statement* (2nd ed). Silver Spring, MD: ANA.

Andrusyszyn, M. A., & Davie, L. (1997). Facilitating reflection through interactive journals writing in an online graduate course: A qualitative study. *Journal of Distance Education, XII*(1/2), 103–126.

Appleton, C. (1994). The gift of self. In P. W. Chin & J. Watson (Eds.), *Art and aesthetics in nursing.* Sudbury, MA: Jones and Bartlett.

Balint, M. (1957). *The doctor, the patient and his illness.* London: Tavistock.

Barrier, P., & Jensen, N. (2003). Two words to improve physician-patient communication: what else? *Mayo Clinic Proceedings, 78*(2), 211–214.

Berry, D. (2006). *Health communication: Theory and practice.* Berkshire, England: Open University Press.

Brennan, A. S. (2006). Theory and practice. In P. D'Antonio, E. Baer, J. Lynaugh, & S. Rinker (Eds.), *Nurse's work.* New York: Springer Publishing Co.

Brykczynski, K. A. (1989). An interpretative study describing the clinical judgment of nurse practitioners. *Scholary Inquiry for Nursing Practice: An International Journal, 3*(2), 75–100.

Chase, S. (2004). *Clinical judgement and communication in nurse practitioner practice.* Philadelphia: F. A. Davis.

Chinn, P. (1994). A method for aesthetic knowing in nursing. In P. W. Chinn (Ed.), *Art & aesthetics in nursing.* New York: National League for Nursing.

Church, O. (1988). Effie J. Taylor. In V. L. Bullough, L. Sentz, O. Maranjian Church, & A. P. Stein (Eds.), *American nursing: A biographical dictionary.* New York: Garland.

Cohen, J., & Welch, L. (2002). Web journaling. Using informational technology to teach reflective practice. *Nursing Leadership Forum,* Summer 6(4), 108–112.

Coulter, A. (1997). Partnerships with patients: The pros and cons of shared clinical decision-making. *Journal of Health Services Research Policy, 2*(2), 112–121.

Crichton, M. (1988). *Travels.* New York: Ballantine Books.

Dolan, J. (1983). *Nursing in society: A historical perspective.* Philadelphia: W.B. Saunders.

Epp, S. (2008). The value of reflective journaling in undergraduate nursing education. *International Journal of Nursing Studies, 45*(9), 1379–1388.

Epstein, R. M., Mauksch, L., Carroll, J. K., & Jaen, C. R. (2008). Have you really addressed your patient's concerns? *Family Practice Management, 15*(3), 35–40.

Fairman, J. (2002). Delegated by default or negotiated by need: Physicians, nurse practitioners, and the process of clinical thinking. In E. Baer, P. D'Antonio, S. Rinker, & J. Lynaugh (Eds.), *Enduring issues in nursing* (pp. 309–333). New York: Springer Publishing Co.

Fawcett, J. (2005). *Contemporary nursing knowledge: Analysis and evaluation of nursing models and theories.* Philadelphia: F.A. Davis Company.

Fenton, M. (1983). Identification of the skilled performance of master's prepared nurses as a method of curriculum planning and evaluation. In P. Benner (Ed.), *From novice to expert: Excellence and power in clinical nursing practice.* Upper Saddle River, NJ: Prentice Hall.

Frankel, R. M., Stein S. T, & Krupat, E. (2003). *The four habits approach to effective clinical communication*. Oakland, CA: The Permanente Medical Group Inc.

Friedman, A. H. (1988). Eufemia A. Taylor. In M. Kaufman (Ed.), *Dictionary of American nursing biography*. Westport, CT: Greenwood.

Green, A. A. (2004). Caring behaviors as perceived by nurse practitioners. *Journal of the American Academy of Nurse Practitioners, 7,* 283–290.

Haag-Heitman, B. (1999). *Clinical practice development: Using novice to expert theory*. Gaithersburg, MD: Aspen Publishers.

Hameric, A., Spross, J., & Hanson, C. (2004). *Advanced practice nursing: An integrative approach* (3rd ed.). Philadelphia: Saunders.

Halva-Neubauer, G. (1995). *Journaling: How it can be a more effective experiential learning technique*. Presented at the annual meeting of the American Political Science Association, New York, NY.

Henderson, V. (1991). *The nature of nursing: Reflections after 25 years*. New York: National League for Nursing Press.

Hiemstra, R. (2001). Uses and benefits of journal writing. In L. M. English & M. A. Gillen (Eds.), *Promoting journal writing in adult education* (New Directions for Adult and Continuing Education, No. 90). San Francisco: Jossey-Bass.

Holmes, S. K., Cramer, I. E., & Charns, M. P. (2003). Becoming patient-centered. *Transition Watch, 6*(3), 3.

Hooker, R. S., Potts, R., & Ray, W. (1997). Patient satisfaction: Comparing physician assistants, nurse practitioners, and physicians. *Permanente Journal, 1* (summer), 5.

Horrocks, S., Anderson, E., & Salisbury, C. (2002). Systematic review of whether nurse practitioners working in primary care can provide equivalent care to doctors. *British Medical Journal, 6,* 5.

Jasper, M. (2003). *Beginning a reflective practice*. Cheltenham: Nelson Thornes.

Jensen, M. (2006). Overview of advanced practice nursing. In M. Jensen & M. Zwygart-Stauffacher (Eds.), *Advanced practice nursing*. New York: Springer Publishing Co.

Johns, C. O. B. P. (2007). Expanding the gates of perception. In C. F. Johns (Ed.), *Transforming nursing through reflective practice*. Oxford: Blackwell Publishing.

Kalisch, P. A., & Kalisch, B. J. (2004). *American nursing: A history* (4th ed.). Philadelphia: Lippincott Williams & Wilkins.

Katz-Wilner, L., & Feinstein-Whittaker, M. (2008, July 27). Career center: optimal patient care. *Advance for Nurse Practitioners*. Retrieved May 8, 2009, from http://nurse-practitioners.advanceweb.com/editorial/content/editorial.aspx?cc=119480&CP=1

Kim, H. S. (1999). Critical reflective inquiry for knowledge development in nursing practice. *Journal of Advanced Nursing, 29*(5), 1205–1212.

King, F. B., & LaRocco, D. J. (2006). E-Journaling: A strategy to support student reflection and understanding. *Current Issues in Education* (online), *9*(4).

Kinnersley, P., Parry, K., Clement, M. J., Archard, L., Turton, P., Stainthorpe, A., et al. (2000). Randomised controlled trial of nurse practitioner versus general practitioner care for patients requesting "same day" consultations in primary care. *British Medical Journal, 16*(Sept), 2.

Lang, F., Floyd, M. R., & Beine, K. L. (2000). Call for active listening. *Archives of Family Medicine, 9,* 222–227.

Laurant, M., Hermens, R., Braspenning, J., Grol, R., & Sibbald, B. (2004). Substitution of doctors by nurses in primary care. *Cochrane Database of Systematic Reviews*, CD001271(4).

Levenstein, J. H., McCracken, S. M., McWhinney, I., Stewart, M., & Brown, J. (1986). The patient-centered clinical method. *Family Practice, 3*, 24–30.

Levinson, W., Roter, D., Mullooly, J., Dull, V., & Frankel, R. (1997). The relationship with malpractice claims among primary care physicians and surgeons. *Journal of American Medical Association, 277*, 553–559.

Lewin, S. A., Entwistle, V., Zwarenstein, M., & Dick, J. (2001). Interventions for providers to promote a patient-centered approach in clinical consultations. *Cochrane Database of Systematic Reviews*, CD003267(4).

Mishler, E. (1984). *Discourse of medicine: Dialectics of medical interviews*. Norwood, NJ: Ablex.

Mok, E., & Chiu, P. C. (2004). Nurse-patient relationships in palliative care. *Journal of Advanced Nursing, 48*(5), 475–483.

Moon, J. (1999). *Learning journals*. London: Kogan Page.

National Association of Clinical Nurse Specialists. (2004). *Statement on Clinical Nurse Specialist practice and education*. Harrisburg, PA: NACNS.

National League for Nursing. (1917). *Standard curriculum for schools of nursing*. New York: NLN.

National League for Nursing. (1936). *Essentials of a good school of nursing*. New York: NLN

National League for Nursing. (1959). *Report on hospital schools of nursing*. New York: NLN.

Neuman, B. & Young, R. (1972). A model for teaching total person approach to patient problems. *Nursing Research, 21*, 264–269.

Oudshoorn, A., Ward-Griffin, C., & McWilliam, C. (2000). Client-nurse relationships in home-based palliative care: a critical analysis of power relations. *Journal of Clinical Nursing, 16*(8), 1435–1443.

Peplau, H. E. (1952). *Interpersonal relations in nursing*. New York: G. P. Putnam's Sons.

Peplau, H. E. (1964). *Basic principles of patient counseling: A conceptual framework of reference for psychodynamic nursing*. New York: Springer Publishing Co.

Pope, E. (1937). *History of nursing education in Texas*. Dallas, TX: Southern Methodist University.

Reiser, D., & Schroder, A. K. (1980). *Patient interviewing: The human dimension*. Baltimore: Williams & Wilkins.

Rosenzweig, M., Hravnak, M., Magdic, K., Beach, M., Clifton, M., & Arnold, R. (2008). Patient communication simulation laboratory for students in an acute care nurse practitioner program. *American Journal of Critical Care, 17*(4), 364–372.

Roter, D. (1989). Which facets of communication have strong effects on outcome: A meta-analysis. In M. Stewart & D. Roter (Eds.), *Communicating with medical patients*. Newbury Park, CA: Sage Publications.

Roter, D., Stewart, M., Putnam, S., Lipkin, M., Stiles, W., & Inui, T. (1997). Communication patterns of primary care physicians. *Journal of American Medical Association, 227*, 350–356.

Schmahl, J. (1966). *Experiment in change: An interdisciplinary approach to the integration of psychiatric content in baccalaureate nursing education*. New York: The Macmillin Company.

Schön, D. (1987, May). *Educating the reflective practitioner*. Paper presented at the American Educational Research Conference, Laramie, WY.

Seale, C., Anderson, E., & Kinnersley, P. (2005). Comparison of GP and nurse practitioner consultations: an observational study. *British Journal of General Practice, 55*(521), 5.

Smith, S. (2006). Clinical decision making in advanced practice nursing. In M. Janson (Ed.), *Advanced practice nursing* (pp. 79–106). New York: Springer Publishing Co.

Sox, H. C. (1979). Quality of patient care by nurse practitioners and physician's assistants: a ten-year perspective. *Annual Internal Medicine, 91*(3), 9.

Stewart, M., Brown, J., Weston, W., McWhinney, I., McWillian, C., & Freeman, T. (1995). *Patient-centered medicine.* Newbury Park, CA: Sage Publications.

Todd, G. (2005). Reflective practice and Socratic dialogue. In C. Johns & D. Freshwater (Eds.), *Transforming nursing through reflective practice.* Hoboken, NJ: Wiley-Blackwell.

Toombs, S. K. (1992). *The meaning of illness: A phenomenological account of the different perspectives of physician and patient.* Norwell, MA: Kluwer Academic Publishers.

Venning, P., Durie, A., Roland, M., Roberts, C., & Leese, B. (2000). Randomised controlled trial comparing cost effectiveness of general practitioners and nurse practitioners in primary care. *British Medical Journal, 320*(7241), 1048–1053.

Williamson, C. (2005). Withholding policies from patients restricts their autonomy. *British Medical Journal, 331*, 1078–1080.

SUGGESTED READINGS

Christy, T. (1969). Portrait of a leader: Isabel Maitland Stewart. *Nursing Outlook, 17*, 44–48.

Donahue, M. P. (1983). Isabel Maitland Stewart's philosophy of education. *Nursing Research, 32*, 140–146.

Hojat, M. (2007). *Empathy in patient care.* New York: Springer Publishing Co.

Swanson, K. M. (1991). Empirical development of a middle-range theory of caring. *Nursing Research, 40,*161–166.

Watson, J. (1988). *Human science and human care: A theory of nursing.* New York: National League for Nursing.

CHAPTER 2

The Healthcare Climate and Communication

Elcha Shain Buckman

People create businesses just like themselves.
People make businesses, businesses don't make people.

—Elcha Shain Buckman

The purpose of this chapter is to examine how healthcare insurance and healthcare delivery systems are affected, influenced, shaped, changed, and transformed by the economy. In order to accomplish this, we will look at both ancient and current history, which has influenced the development of medicine and our healthcare delivery system. The existing economic climate, which interfaces with political and medical structures, will continue to change and, therefore, affect the design of these systems of care. We will examine what the future holds and how prevailing influences might affect clinical practice and patient care. All of these issues demand attention to issues related to communication. Finally, specific exercises will facilitate realistic application of theory to practice.

HISTORICAL BACKGROUND

A More Current Event

History is a vast early warning system.

—Norman Cousins

When applied to health care, this statement indicates that the best way to even hope to understand the present healthcare climate and steward its direction is to know the history of the gargantuan and transformational changes that have happened to the world in general and in the US healthcare delivery system in particular, especially since the early 1900s.

If you don't know where you're going you might wind up someplace else.
When you come to a fork in the road, take it.
It ain't over till it's over.
I never said most of the things I said.

—Yogi Berra

These seminal statements, known as Yogiisms, made by an eighth grade educated, 1940s great and most beloved New York Yankees' baseball catcher and manager, have been embraced by the businesspeople (yes, men and women alike) throughout the United States, particularly when they cannot think of another way to express their feelings.

These Yogiisms unfortunately can also describe what has become our present economic crisis and current state of US healthcare delivery systems. Since 1935 and the advent of Social Security, there exists a confusing mixture of health insurance products and services. Today there are over a dozen different types of delivery systems for health care, and universal health care may be on the horizon.

A Little Ancient History

"Above all else, do no harm," a common phrase when talking about patients and health care, is attributed to Hippocrates (b. 460 BC), the father of medicine. It is said to be from his famous Hippocratic Oath (a code of ethics for physicians) which is still taken by many modern medical, dental, and nursing school graduates around the world. In fact, "Above all else, do no harm" does not appear in The Hippocratic Oath. The confusion may have arisen from the fact that, during the time of Hippocrates, doctors used to administer (for a price) fatal potions to dispatch unwanted individuals to their heavenly reward. Hippocrates strongly disapproved of this practice and did include the phrase "I will neither give a deadly drug to anybody if asked for it, nor will I make a suggestion to this effect" (Temkin & Temkin, 1967). This cryptic saying effectively conveys the Hippocratic principles. Hippocrates, history's most famous physician, is best known for what today would be referred to as *patient-centered care*. He rejected superstition, which was the prevailing medical practice in terms of both diagnostics and treatment at the time. Rather, he classified diseases according to scientific observation and created moral and professional standards for physicians. His innovations were so revolutionary and held in such high esteem that virtually no significant medical and healthcare discoveries occurred until 1135 and the birth of Maimonides. This world-renowned Jewish physician was also a rabbi, religious scholar, philosopher, mathematician, and astronomer. Like Hippocrates, his life was entirely focused on improving health conditions and patient care while changing health behaviors and laws. His best known writing is his collection of medical aphorisms: *Treatise on Poisons and their Antidotes, Treatise on Hemorrhoids, Treatise on Cohabitation, Treatise on the Regimen of Health, Treatise on the Causes of Symptoms, Laws of Human Temperaments,* and *Treatise on Asthma.* Such works have been translated by Jewish medical ethicist Fred Rosner (Battista & McCabe, 1999). In his famous *The Guide for the Perplexed Maimonides,* he provides the view that the ancient Israelite food laws and actions have health benefits and purpose. This work directly led to health food laws, such as kosher dietary laws, and was later adopted by Islam as halal and progressively adopted worldwide.

Not-So-Ancient History

In 1883, poet Emma Lazarus wrote the sonnet *The New Colossus* which was later engraved on the plaque affixed to the lobby of the Statue of Liberty in New York Harbor at its dedication in 1886. The most recognized portion of the sonnet is:

> *Give me your tired, your poor, Your huddled masses yearning to breathe free, The wretched refuse of your teeming shore. Send these, the homeless, tempest-tost to me.*

This poem was written on the pedestal of the Statue of Liberty. It is the most recognized symbol of freedom in the world. It might seem strange to include a poet as an influence on our present day healthcare climate, but her words have not only become a cornerstone in the foundation of our caring about freedom, but have become a commitment for freedom for all people and a cornerstone in our commitment to their health care as well. However, it is Hippocrates whose name and admonishment endures for all healthcare providers: Above all else, do no harm.

Up to Date

It is the likes of Hippocrates, Maimonides, and Lazarus of our medical and world history who posthumously and most significantly resonate for healthcare practitioners; their influence is seen in reflective practice as identified by Harry S.

Sullivan (1953) and Martin Buber (1970); provider–patient relationships as written about by Hildegard Peplau (1952), Ida Jean Orlando (1961), and Elcha Shain Buckman (1994); and self-appreciation espoused by H. L. Dreyfus and S. E. Dreyfus (1986) and Patricia Benner (1984). US citizens are proud of their expansive healthcare system and its expertly prepared advanced healthcare practitioners. Immigrants (legal and illegal) and visitors from abroad have always come to the United States for the opportunities provided by our healthcare delivery systems, freedoms, earning power, and education systems that they and their families can participate and share in. What has previously been the most respected and sought-after healthcare system worldwide, US health care and its multiple choice delivery systems are beginning to disappoint and lag behind other countries, wealthy and poor. Some recent history of the development of our modern yet somewhat flagging healthcare system will bring this into perspective.

Social Security was established as law in 1935 but did not include any healthcare provisions because physician and insurance company lobbies kept them out. It was not until the United States' transition to the Information Age (late 1950s) from the Industrial Era (late 1800s and early 1900s) that the economy began to play a powerful role in shaping the healthcare climate for US citizens and immigrants. Healthcare laws, such as Medicare and Medicaid in 1965, and other economic laws affecting health care, such as the Omnibus Reconciliation Act of 1990 and the Balanced Budget Act of 1997 which included the Children's Health Insurance Program, were created. Coincidentally, from the early 1960s, health care became hostage to the collateral damage of big business forcing the transition from a private-payer system to multipayer and managed care systems and from a medical art and science service industry to a mostly medical science and medico-technology business.

In the late 1970s, healthcare providers were discussing not *whether* medicine was going from high-touch/low-tech to low-touch/high-tech, but *when*. In February 2009, days after his inauguration, President Obama, along with all media outlets and headlines, drove home the messages of economic recession and financial crisis in insurance coverage and medical services.

US health care has been living well for 40 years, but after 50 years of healthcare reform we are on life support. There is continuous threatening talk of Social Security and Medicare running out of money by 2020. On February 24, 2009, President Obama announced a $643 billion bailout for health care over the next 10 years. Hope is high, but the prognosis is extremely grave.

At the beginning of the 21st century, providers find our practice and the system of delivering health care bound to current, yet rapidly changing, economic and political realities. The US healthcare climate has become a conundrum of advancing medical diagnostics, treatments, pharmaceuticals, technologies, and research. For a list of healthcare terms and definitions see Box 2-1.

Box 2-1 Frequently Used Healthcare Delivery Systems Terms and Definitions

Bottom line	The end result of an analysis; usually refers to financials; can refer to the profit realized by the company.
Beds	Up to 25% more than the actual number of bed capacity in any given hospital.
Capitation	After complex cost/benefit and risk analysis based on the number of patients listed with the health maintenance organization (HMO) by the provider, this is the flat-fee payment by the insurer to the contracted provider, without regard to actual health service needs. When a patient requires higher than average level of care, the patient's provider must absorb the extra cost. Conversely, when the lower than average level of care is required, the provider absorbs the savings. This creates financial incentives for the provider to limit care options offered to patients and to shun patients with complex needs while trying to attract young, healthier patients.
The Centers for Medicare and Medicaid Services (CMS)	The government administrators, approvers, and financial overseers of Medicare and Medicaid providers and patient claims.
Cost/Benefit ratio (C/B)	Used in capital budgeting; the formula used to control costs which tells the insurer if they are getting the most from each medical service for every dollar spent; the relationship considered in the analysis of whether the benefit is worth, or greater than, the cost of the medical intervention.
Formulary	A multitiered prescription program identifying the cost of medications according to the designated areas in which they fall: generic, nonpreferred, and preferred, from the cheapest to the most expensive.

Box 2-1 Frequently Used Healthcare Delivery Systems Terms and Definitions *(continued)*

Heads	The numbers of individuals receiving care in a hospital, outpatient, or clinic setting; the number of patients a primary care provider carries as a caseload, as dictated by the HMO with whom that provider has a reimbursement contract; used when referring to capitation.
Healthcare Delivery System	Any insurer, company, or business entity that pays or reimburses a licensed practitioner for providing medical services to a patient; coverage and reimbursement based on a complex internal system of policies, procedures, and finances.
The Health Insurance Portability and Accountability Act (HIPAA)	Defines the standards for electronic healthcare transactions and patient privacy.
Managed care	An organization that has a paid arrangement for providing health care in which the organization acts as an intermediary between the person seeking care and the physician and providers of other healthcare services; the for-profit side of the business of providing health care to people.
Panel	A provider who is an accepted member of a managed care organization's network.
Preapproved	The approval by the insurer for a medically necessary patient treatment, which must be given before the treatment is administered.
Perqs	Corporate perquisites; benefits provided by an employer to its employees.

Advances in imaging procedures, surgery, and pharmaceuticals are driving up the cost of health care. As the population ages, additional demands will be placed on the system. Increasingly influential and complex lobbying and political systems (some physicians and nurses are now state and national legislators) and permanently powerful financial institutions and investment houses have all become crucial partners in the business of health care.

What would be termed modern and reformed health care began its move in the early 1900s and has pretty much stalled early in the 21st century. What began as an exclusively US, single-payer, private indemnity insurance-based healthcare delivery system has ended in a morass of multipayer, managed healthcare systems. We have shifted from a blue-collar, agricultural–industrial society to a more educated, white-collar, global, and technological society. Health care has shifted from patient-centered care as might be described by Harry S. Sullivan (1953), Carl Rogers (1951), Hildegard Peplau (1952), Ida Jean Orlando (1961), and Elcha Shain Buckman (1994), to economic-centered patient care as determined by Kaiser-Permanente, CIGNA, Tenent, Pacificare, UnitedHealthcare, and Humana.

THE BUSINESS OF US HEALTHCARE: A RESPONSE TO CHANGE

US Healthcare Insurance Models

We are the prisoners of history. Or are we?

—Robert Penn Warren, *Segregation*

No matter what we are told, the present US healthcare insurance industry is not market driven. The development of our healthcare delivery models are designed in response to (1) the current healthcare business climate, (2) the country's prevailing economic situation, and (3) the expectations of its citizens. Therefore, the US healthcare insurance industry can be said to be product driven and/or economy driven. The focus here will be on a review of the development, types, and components of our healthcare delivery models; a review of our unique US healthcare climate as influenced by the design of a prevailing business (i.e., the insurance industry, its healthcare models, and delivery systems); and the effect on and affect by the prevailing economic climate. Later in this chapter we will look at how today's healthcare climate can be affected, controlled, and influenced by communication and what types of communication and actions are needed to make changes for the better.

HEALTH CARE TRANSFORMED: 1935 TO 1980

History is the sum total of the things that could have been avoided.

—Konrad Adenauer

Corporate perquisites (perqs) were the first health insurance products. In the early 1900s, during World War I, the United States entered the Industrial Era, bringing with it labor unions and increasing corporate responsibilities to and for its employees. The company owners, executives, and board members could easily afford to pay for their health care. Other employees, or line workers, were over worked, under paid, and had no to little access to health care.

Labor unions originated to support line workers and, as such, were and historically remain at odds with management, which is made up of executive (referred to as C level, such as in chief operating officer), management, and supervisory level employees. The rest of the employees, line workers, referred to the importance of manufacturing and products produced in a line. With the advent of labor unions, basic line employees began to see improved working conditions (lighting, air, breaks) and safety improvements, some attention to the health of workers, better pay, a 40-hour work week and overtime pay, child labor laws, and job security. Corporations rewarded loyal workers by giving them regular pay increases, overtime pay, vacation time and pay, and paid for their healthcare costs and provided on-site or neighborhood clinics or provided in-house doctors and nurses who were available during working hours.

Some companies purchased policies covering limited health care. The first insurance plans were administered by new, private insurance companies such as Sears and John Hancock. Line worker employees, in turn, rewarded employers by being hard working, conscientious, reliable, and loyal. Particularly with health care covered, even to a limited extent, loyalty was so high that certain industries like manufacturing or coal mining were known to have multiple, successive generations working for them. Changed labor laws and accompanying healthcare provisions and policies of the late 19th century gave birth to private indemnity insurance, often referred to as 80/20 because 80% of the healthcare bill was paid by the insurance company and 20% was paid by the individual for any and all healthcare services, from doctor's office visits to hospital stays. This system is the original comprehensive healthcare insurance; it can still be found but to a much lesser extent. Private indemnity was the sole type of private healthcare insurance until the 1930s when Kaiser-Permanente, a private HMO, focused on prevention (see HMO section later). The 70 years of coverage by private indemnity insurance policies were also the years that physicians controlled, managed, and led health care and hospitals. These halcyon years provided unprecedented financial prosperity with minimal interference in medical decision making by the payers. During this time, medicine and healthcare services were considered an art and science.

Now that the healthcare climate is a managed care business climate, the private indemnity insurance market share has been reduced to approximately 15%. However, the sales of HMOs' point of service (POS) health insurance plans (see later discussion) and health savings accounts (HSAs) are on the rise. These appear to have structured themselves similarly to parts of private indemnity policies.

The US stock market crashed on October 24, 1929, a day known as Black Thursday. Thousands of people lost nearly or their entire investments with many bankers committing suicide. The losses continued into the following Tuesday. Black Tuesday, October 29, 1929, was the start of the Great Depression, which lasted nearly a decade. Massive levels of poverty, hunger, unemployment, and political unrest followed and spread to Europe and the rest of the world. In an effort to provide financial support for the unemployed, and as a stop-gap measure for poverty and hunger to ever recur, the Social Security Act was ratified on August 14, 1935 by President Franklin D. Roosevelt. Social Security, a uniquely American solution, was established as a system of old-age and disability benefits, becoming the foundation for the establishment of Medicare in 1965 and Medicaid in 1966. Social Security does not require mandatory retirement at any age, but the age of eligibility is reviewed and reset periodically higher by the government. This enables Social Security to be maintained by keeping employment contributions coming in.

The amount one collects in annual Social Security is determined by how many quarters they contribute while working. The maximum of 40 quarters is then calculated on the highest income one earned for those 40 quarters. An individual of retirement age can elect to forego collecting Social Security and continue working and contribute to Social Security until they choose to retire. Opposition by the medical profession and private insurance interests kept health insurance out of the Social Security Act of 1935. Medicare and Medicaid (see following text) were ratified in 1965 and went into effect in 1966, becoming an intrinsic component of our national welfare system. After 30 years of going through various amendments and bitter disagreements, it was clear that health insurance needed to be enacted. The major issues were whether the program would be compulsory or voluntary, serve all incomes or just the poor, and be run by the federal government or the states; also at issue was how public and private agencies would be balanced. The ratified 1965 amendment to the Social Security Act was a compromise: Medicare would be federally run and serve the elderly and disabled of all incomes; Medicaid would serve the poor and be state administered. Medicare is solely a federal trust fund for working US citizens, whose funds are collectable upon retirement. Medicare was originally made up of Part A as mandatory coverage for hospitalization, and Part B as optional coverage that may be deferred if the beneficiary or their spouse is still actively working. There is a lifetime penalty (10% per year) imposed for not enrolling in Part B unless actively working (Kung, Hoyert, Xu, & Murphy, 2008).

The Medicare trust fund is administered by CMS, a component of the Department of Health and Human Services (HHS) in concert with other federal financial departments. In 2007, Medicare provided healthcare coverage for 43 million of the US population, with enrollment expected to reach 77 million by

2031 when the baby boom generation is fully enrolled. Each employee contributes 2.9% of their earnings annually—half by the employee and half from the employer. Medicare was established as a two-part system, Part A (federally funded insurance) and Part B (individually purchased supplemental insurance).

According to the Medicare Information Center, the annual cost of Medicare Part A is prorated on a monthly basis and the amount is deducted from each person's monthly Social Security check. In 2009, that deduction is $96.40 a month which, under Part A, covers limited financial benefits and stays, or both, in hospital, home health, hospice, and skilled nursing facilities (SNFs). Medicare recipients must meet a yearly deductible before Medicare coverage begins. People who have the financial ability can purchase Part B, a private supplementary insurance policy to cover or assist with what costs remain of Part A as the patient's responsibility, covers almost all other necessary medical services including office visits, treatments, and diagnostic tests. A convoluted Part D, purchased separately, became law in 2003 providing limited, proscribed financial assistance with selected prescription drugs, according to a formulary. For individuals who choose an HMO as their supplemental insurance, Part B and Part D become Part C (Medicare choice). In most instances, the monthly $96.40 deduction is the capitation cost for Part C. Medigap is the identifying name and is the federal supplemental equivalent of Medicare for low-income, retired, Medicaid-eligible clients. Permanent Medicaid disability (Supplemental Security Income [SSI]) is converted to Medicare after 2 years and can, in this instance, be collected before full retirement age. In 1965, federal retirement was set at age 65 and was mandatory in most companies; hence, the storied gold watch given at retirement when 65 years old. In 1978 pressure from activist groups, particularly the Gray Panthers, changed the mandatory retirement age from 65 to 70 years old. The Medicare program made a significant step for social welfare legislation and helped establish the growing population of elderly as a pressure group. In 1965, 3.9 million Americans were receiving Medicare benefits and the expected average life span was 68.5 years old for men and 72 years old for women, with 14- to 21-year-olds as the fastest growing segment of the population. The much improved quality of medical care and technological advances have increased life expectancies. In 2005, 50 million Americans were Medicare beneficiaries and the expected life span was 75.2 years for men and 80.4 years for women, with people older than the age of 100 being the fastest growing segment of the population (Ridgway, 2008).

A look at life expectancies, based on the last census taken in 2005, is revealing. It is projected that, in 2010, 70 million Americans will be covered by Medicare and the United States will have a population of 310.3 billion people, growing to 341.4 billion in 2020. The Medicare eligibility age was raised in 2000 from 65 to 67 years old. These foregoing statistics have enormous implications for Medicare and all other healthcare providers and insurers.

The political and financial designers of Medicare were unable to anticipate its present evolution. To lower costs the government periodically redefines retirement age and adds other legislation, thereby enabling the longevity of our Medicare trust fund. Contracted Medicare providers are paid for their services according to the usual and customary charges in their geographical area. The recent additions of HMO-managed Medicare and Part D have severely worsened an already perplexing healthcare climate, to say nothing about the extraordinary lack of public information and understanding. In 1965, prescription medication coverage was not the issue it has become today. Prescribed drugs were given to the patient by the physician who had well-stocked samples from drug representatives and prescriptions were relatively inexpensive to fill.

Since the 1980s, innovative and sophisticated pharmaceutical research and development, pioneering medical technology, reduced coverage by HMOs, and pharmaceutical manufacturers' increased mass marketing and advertising of new and expensive prescription drugs to the public have triggered unbridled rising medication costs for consumers. In 2003 a well-meaning effort to relieve the health-insured consumer of exorbitant medication costs, President George W. Bush complicated the situation by creating and signing into law a convoluted Medicare Part D—incomprehensible to all, even the insurers. In the arena of political healthcare football, many politicians warn of the government's inability to continue Medicare coverage after 2020. From a business standpoint, Medicare, as a healthcare delivery system, is reasonably well organized and is a relatively financially well-managed insurer. Some who are active and knowledgeable in the financial, business, and healthcare industries posit that if universal healthcare coverage is adopted by the federal government then it should be designed like the Medicare/Medicaid model and managed by CMS. These and other proposals to expand competition in (and out of) Medicare are controversial because they are based more on theory than on practice generating apprehension about the risks to beneficiaries. Until then, or until health care and insurance services and costs are strategically investigated and restructured, Medicare will remain only one part of our tangled healthcare quagmire.

Medicaid was instituted in 1966 and is currently the largest healthcare insurer in the United States. It is jointly administered by federal and state governments under Title XIX of the Social Security Act. Medicaid was preceded by the Kerr-Mills Act of 1960, which provided federal support for state medical programs serving the elderly poor. Because the passage of the Kerr-Mills Act and Medicare preceded it, Medicaid was easily passed by Congress but has become the government's most expensive general welfare program. Although state participation in Medicaid is voluntary, all states have participated since 1982. The federal government reimburses states according to per capita income, with states like New York receiving 50 cents and Mississippi receiving 80 cents for every dollar spent on Medicaid. According to CMS, in 2004, Medicaid payments totaled $295 billion. To help defray rapidly rising costs, a new federal rule was passed on November 25, 2008, that allowed states to charge premiums and higher copayments to Medicaid recipients. The mission of Medicaid is to provide the over 55 million disabled, elderly, low-income, and poverty-level US citizens and resident aliens with access to private-equivalent levels of normal medical health care, including dental care and prescription drug rebates. Medicaid covers in-hospital, SNF, out-patient, and office care. Statistics point to Medicaid enrollment being mostly single women with children (60%), the disabled (20%), and poor elderly (20%) with dual Medicare and Medicaid eligibility. Under federal law, states cannot reduce welfare benefits when individuals become Medicaid eligible. All Medicaid payments are made to providers only and this has created Medicaid's major problem: fraud. Although some successful reforms have been instituted, other problems still persist (Box 2-2).

Medicaid suffers from the same issues and problems as Medicare and all other healthcare insurers: rising costs of health care, increase in eligible individuals, increased use of services by individuals, movement from fee-for-service to managed care contracts compromising assurance of standards of care, stagnation of quality of the health care provided, and expansion of what is considered minimum benefits.

The years after World War II ushered in even more extraordinary advances in the ability of medical care to prevent and relieve suffering through the research and development of powerful diagnostic tools and sophisticated treatments and

---

Box 2-2 Problems with Medicaid

Being state administered, the quality and range of medical services varies considerably
Because services are contracted with private payers, costs cannot be easily controlled
Because illegal immigrants qualify in many circumstances, this puts extra care and cost burdens on certain states
Hospital emergency rooms are financially vulnerable because illegal immigrants are covered for emergency services
Childless couples and single adults who live at low-income or poverty levels are not covered unless disabled

medicines. We had the polio vaccine and immunosuppressants; we began using computed tomography (CT) scans, positron emission tomography (PET) scans, and magnetic resonance imaging (MRI); we discovered that a naturally occurring water-soluble salt called lithium was the rescue treatment for people suffering from manic-depressive illness; and open-heart surgery, kidney dialysis machines, and organ transplants were saving hundreds of thousands of lives a year. In 1900, the average life expectancy in the United States was 47 years and the major causes of death each year were various infections. By the late 1940s, because of the development of highly developed life support systems, powerful antibiotics, and corticosteroids, chronic diseases such as cancer, stroke, and heart attacks had replaced infections as the major causes of death and, toward the end of the 20th century, life expectancy in the United States had increased to 87 years. Some Americans are now called the *sandwich* generation because they are taking care of their children and their parents now coping with Alzheimer's disease, the scourge of modern medicine, or cancer and dementia. Exceptional scientific advancements, along with the Civil Rights movement, have resulted in profound changes in the US healthcare system. Before World War II most physicians were general practitioners and by 1960, almost 90% chose careers in a specialty area. Solo practice faded and physicians began group practices. Health care became more of right for all citizens, thus increasing the numbers who sought care.

Social and healthcare reforms, Social Security, and Medicare ended segregation in hospitals. Private medical insurance companies, including Blue Cross/Blue Shield, Aetna, and Fireman's Fund, began to offer health insurance to the middle class. Prosperity followed for both providers and hospitals. Medical specialization flourished and yet care became ever more fragmented. Research and technological advances raised ethical issues while disease prevention and health promotion were ignored. Paperwork and red tape began to clog the system. Soaring costs became the major concern, dwarfing the concern about the uninsured and the issue of access to care.

Employers began to realize that their competitiveness in the global market was being lost to foreign companies that paid far less for employee health insurance than they did, and employees feared losing healthcare benefits because of jobs being sent overseas.

The Era of Managed Care: 1985 to Present

This era of rapidly progressing technology advances came roaring on the national scene like a pride of lions in the early 1980s, revolutionizing the field of medical science, research, development, and services in every way possible—

many of which have been welcomed changes. Following this, the cost of health care began soaring out of control in the mid-1980s. In addition, the medical profession's and federal regulator's inability to control costs, combined for a business-imposed approach of *managed care* to take over, resulting in the new business of health care. Managed care is a generic term that refers to a large variety of reimbursement plans in which third-party payers attempt to control costs by limiting the utilization of medical services, in contrast to the hands-off style of traditional fee-for-service payment. Included in this permanent change to healthcare services are:

1. Prescribing medications according to a formulary
2. Mandating preauthorizations before treatments, procedures, surgeries, and hospitalizations are provided
3. Severely restricting the length of time a patient may remain in the hospital and requiring that patients be allowed to see specialists only if referred by a *gatekeeper* (the primary care physician or the insurance company)

Some of these changes have had positive outcomes, while others are not without their disadvantages (Table 2-1).

What was first proffered as innovative systems of delivering cost-effective health care quickly became recognized as profit-motivated, investor-owned organizations. So it appears that managed care has unfortunately ushered in a new era of significant vocal public backlash against it and strident patients' rights advocacy. Perqs continue to live and be well and play a stronger role than ever in businesses large and small. As employees, we are a society used to our employer paying for our healthcare insurance (and our family's) since the 1950s; as retirees, we are used to them continuing to pay and provide until we and our spouse die. Or, we expect the same from Medicare. The hottest topics constantly and consistently talked about since 2004 are:

1. Will the company be able to continue to provide healthcare coverage for its working employees? And, if so, what percentage will the company and employee each pay?
2. How can the company legally get out of paying for the healthcare coverage promised to their retirees?
3. Medicare is in a crisis; it is assumed that the government only has money to cover until 2020; the recessive economy (with unemployment and bankruptcies at their highest rate ever recorded) is not allowing for the coffers to continue to be filled. How long will the money really last and how long can it continue to cover today's and tomorrow's retirees?

How's that for the healthcare climate and communication!

Table 2-1 Advantages and Disadvantages of Managed Care

Advantages
Patients are now consumers, leading to such things as better hospital food, previously thought of as complaining or irrelevant
Respect, recognition, and expansion of services by advanced practice nurses and pharmacists
Creation and growth of physician extender programs (physician assistants and medical technicians)
Efficiency of information technologies, providing confidentiality and saving time and space for people, offices, and institutions
The medical profession thinking seriously about costs
Some treatments and procedures safely moved from hospitals to less costly ambulatory settings
Improved business practices regarding healthcare delivery system
Disadvantages
In spite of, or because of, advanced technology, utilization review, and preauthorization there has been a serious erosion of the quality of our health care
A serious loss of trust in doctors and our healthcare system
Triple-digit healthcare inflation
It has not been able to keep its promise of controlling healthcare costs
The *dollar-is-king* and *medicine-is-a-marketplace* business mentality has been seriously detrimental to some areas of healthcare services, medical schools, and teaching hospitals

Health Maintenance Organizations (Managed Care)

All providers must be contracted with the HMO and must accept their capitation rules. HMOs are organized around the following assumption: Control costs by paying less for fewer services. The underlying tenets are stringent utilization review, cost reduction by reimbursing providers less for services, cost containment by allowing referrals only to in-plan providers, and preauthorization for all procedures and treatments other than in clear emergency situations. In the United States, HMOs caused the demise of virtually all private payer insurances. As much as we may rail against it, we have socialized medicine and it is called HMO. And, we have had it as our major third-party payer since 1980. Socialized medicine is defined as a government-regulated system for providing health care for all by means of subsidies derived from taxation. Universal health care (see later discussion) is defined as healthcare coverage (including medical, dental, and mental health care), which vary in their structure and funding mechanisms and is extended to all eligible residents of a governmental region. With universal health care, typically most costs are met via a single-payer healthcare system or compulsory health insurance. Universal health care is provided in all wealthy, industrialized countries except for the United States and in many developing countries, and is the trend worldwide.

Ironically, the first HMO, nonprofit Kaiser Permanente, had been organized in the 1930s to achieve better coordination and continuity of care and to emphasize preventive medical services. Any cost savings that were achieved were considered a secondary benefit. By the 1980s, however, the attempt to control costs had become the dominant force underlying the managed care movement. HMOs were the new insurance of and for the Information Age. They promised reduced annual policy costs and large cost savings through better utilization of medical services, focus on prevention, and improved management of the healthcare dollar. These promises have not been realized. In fact, since the take over by HMOs, the cost of their annual insurance policies (along with the cost of health care) tripled by 2005.

What first started as merger and management of physician group practices quickly evolved into the addition and management of many healthcare facilities, satellite clinics, and some hospitals and, subsequently, the purchase, control, and restructuring of healthcare insurance companies. So began the era of managing and controlling healthcare delivery systems and healthcare dollars. In 1969, Harvard Community Health Plan (HCHP), established in Boston, fashioned itself after Kaiser-Permanente. Both plans were developed to provide in-house employee health care: Kaiser-Permanente in 1945 for the vast California healthcare system and HCHP for Harvard University and its teaching hospitals' students, staff and faculty, and their families. Kaiser-Permanente, expanding to include other West Coast states, continues to exist as a strong West Coast nonprofit HMO. HCHP, however, after rapid growth to include many off-site health centers, did not fair as well. The 1970s ushered in the age of medical technology and the rapid increase of the cost of health care. This worsening and grossly expensive healthcare climate led to the rise of other HMOs across the country, believing and selling the idea that they could slow the runaway train. In Boston, other universities with medical schools, such a Tufts, competed by establishing their own internal HMO systems. For a short time, in the late 1970s, the HCHP acronym became loosely known in the Boston healthcare community as Horrible Care for Health People—referring to the decline of their services as it grew through merger and acquisition to include other HMO healthcare delivery systems outside of the huge Harvard University umbrella. In the late 1990s, HCHP was acquired by Pilgrim Health Care, a Boston-based HMO corporation and renamed Harvard-Pilgrim, a for-profit HMO. Across the country, the late 1970s and even 1980s brought the injudicious growth of HMOs (many lawyer-owned for financial expediency and later found to be illegal), especially in the South. Many HMOs became publically owned companies, run by high-paid executives, and, as public companies, were responsible to their stock- and stakeholders first, their contracted providers second, and their contracted customers, the patients, last.

As large companies, HMOs only contract with large groups—businesses, physician groups, healthcare facilities, Medicare, and Medicaid. The bottom-line profit and rising stock prices became primary, and healthcare delivery became secondary. These HMOs became known as cash cows for their owners and executives, and a scourge for physicians who were being financially deprived and professionally controlled through sharply reduced fees paid for preapproved procedures and corporate denial of many usual and customary procedures. Today's patients, who are more educated, informed, and involved in their healthcare decisions, are complaining as well of experiencing a decline in healthcare services, an increase in copayments for preapproved services, and the rising cost of their annual healthcare policies. At the same time, employers are cutting back coverage and the portion they pay of the annual policies, thereby increasing the percentage employees pay for their annual policies. Clearly, we have gotten the message that HMOs are not the answer to our healthcare climate dilemmas. Since the inception of HMOs, recurring incidences of corporate fraud, widespread merger and acquisition activity, pervasive misuse of patient records by healthcare and insurance corporations and some employers, and invasive violations of human rights led to the creation and establishment of HIPAA (see later discussion).

Preferred/Participating Provider Organizations

A preferred/participating provider organization (PPO) is a second, less managed, more expensive managed care organization of medical doctors, hospitals, and other healthcare providers who have contracted with an insurer or HMO as a third-party administrator to provide health care at reduced rates. It allows more flexibility of choice in providers and services than an HMO. A PPO earns money by charging an access fee to the third-party administrator for the use of their network, allowing insurance companies to negotiate directly with hospitals and physicians for health services at a lower price than would be normally charged. PPOs employ the same utilization review procedures to verify that the recommended procedures or treatments are appropriate for the condition being treated, as well as a near-universal precertification requirement for everything other than emergency services.

PPOs try to combine the best elements of a fee-for-service and an HMO. A PPO provides the subscriber with a greater selection of healthcare service providers—in most cases not requiring a primary care physician referral—and can be viewed as a more traditional plan that uses discounted fees as the cost savings to the managed care company and a perceived increase in services by the subscriber.

Since the proliferation of HMOs and PPOs, the competitive advantages over POS and private indemnity insurance have largely been reduced or almost entirely eliminated. This accounts for medical inflation in the United States again advancing at 150 to 200% the rate of general inflation. Furthermore, the aspects of utilization review and precertification are now widely used even in traditional private indemnity plans, and are widely regarded as being essentially permanent features of the US healthcare system.

Point of Service Insurance

POS plans are a third, most expensive version of an HMO. The POS plan offers two options for the delivery of health care: (1) An open access network allowing the subscriber the right to select a provider within the HMO whenever care is needed without the intervention of a gatekeeper. This option will have a higher physician copayment than its traditional HMO counterpart and may require a deductible as well, plus a designated percentage as a co-insurance requirement. (2) An out-of-network option permits the subscriber to choose a provider outside the HMO network at the time care is required and there is no gatekeeper/director. This option has a high deductible (perhaps $500 or more) before payment is made to a provider for service and an 80/20 co-insurance requirement until the enrollee's out-of-pocket medical expenses reach a high annual deductible (usually $5000), and then the plan would pay all expenses up to a lifetime maximum ($750,000 to $1,000,000).

The Health Insurance Portability and Accountability Act

HIPAA was enacted by the US Congress in 1996. According to the CMS Web site, Title I of HIPAA protects health insurance coverage for workers and their families when they change or lose their jobs. Title II of HIPAA, known as the Administrative Simplification (AS) provisions, requires the establishment of national standards for electronic healthcare transactions and national identifiers for providers, health insurance plans, and employers. The AS provisions also address the security and privacy of health data. The standards are meant to improve the efficiency and effectiveness of the nation's healthcare system by encouraging the widespread use of an electronic data interchange in the US healthcare system.

Catastrophic Health Insurance Plans

Also known as high deductible health plans (HDHPs), catastrophic health insurance plans (CHIPs) were created as a way to lower overall medical costs by providing a lower monthly premium in exchange for a higher annual health insurance deductible. With CHIPs, you pay for almost all medical care until you reach the annual deductible amount (usually $25,000). After that, traditional, 80/20 private indemnity health insurance coverage begins. If the CHIP is eligible for an HSA, the subscriber can use the funds contributed to help defray the deductible and out-of-pocket expenses. CHIPs have high lifetime maximum benefit payment limits (also known as caps), usually between $1 million and $5 million. Once the cap has been reached, the health insurance company will not pay for any of the subscriber's medical costs and the policy will be cancelled. These health insurance plans can usually be purchased either as an individual plan or as a group, but are very stringent about not covering preexisting conditions. The most common reasons for choosing a CHIP are: (1) you are young and would rather risk getting sick than pay high premiums for full coverage plans, even HMOs; (2) you have enough money to pay for all of your regular health care including short-term surgery and/or hospitalizations; (3) you would use it as a supplementary policy to provide choice of healthcare providers around the world; and (4) you want sufficient coverage for the catastrophic costs associated with diseases such as cancer.

Healthcare Savings Account

This type of healthcare coverage plan is becoming increasingly popular for self-employed individuals and small businesses. As the numbers of unemployed, bankruptcies, and personal and corporate spending cutbacks increase in the recessive 2009 economic climate, it stands to reason that the numbers of HSAs will increase along with the Medicaid roles. HSAs are tax-exempt, tax-deductible ways of saving for the costs of illnesses. There are no withdrawal requirements except that the employee must use the money only for health care. Some believe, especially young healthy people, that it is smart to set aside some money each month to pay for future medical expenses that you may incur, even if you do not use the money until later in life. Personal responsibility and choice are the key concepts upon which this type of healthcare benefits plan is predicated. An HSA is exactly as it states: a personal cash savings account established by an individual or through his/her company, which is designated solely for the purpose of drawing on these monies to pay for health care. Each state differs in guidelines and tax benefits; certain state and nationally determined tax deductions and/or nontaxable benefits exist. Some states also set an annual minimum balance that must be maintained and/or minimum annual contributions made to the account. An HSA can be established separately along with a CHIP to provide for broader and more comprehensive coverage. The thinking behind this type of nontraditional healthcare savings and payment system is to provide freedom of choice of physicians, treatments, procedures, medications, and healthcare facilities and hospitals. Many physicians, pharmacies, hospitals, and healthcare facilities will provide discounts for services if they are being paid from the accumulated cash in a HSA.

Boutique Physician Practices

These practices are also called concierge, elite, premium, even platinum, practices. Once the pariah of medicine because of its seeming elitist, country club, only-the-wealthy-could-afford aura, boutique practices are now a viable choice for many. Since 2007, there have been continuing education courses designed for physicians, nurse practitioners, and physician assistants to learn the practicalities and legalities of opening boutique practices. Today there are hundreds of physicians in private concierge-type practices. These practices are a response to the confines and restrictions of managed care organizations. Having been a patient for 12 years, your author was one of the first patients in the second-ever boutique practice, started by Robert Colton, MD, in Boca Raton, Florida, in 2000 under the name MDVIP (the first boutique practice, MD2, opened in Seattle, WA, in 1996). MDVIP is now a successful organization with member physicians in 23 states. Since 2000, boutique practices have been started by other physicians independently.

Boutique practices began as a reclaiming by one physician of his professional, and personal, life from the control and dictates of managed care organizations. Physicians open concierge practices as a way of escaping managed care for these reasons:

1. Their incomes have been threatened and compromised.
2. Utilization review, preauthorization, required large caseloads, capitation, and paperwork have severely injured and compromised their ability to provide a high quality of care.
3. To have a personal life. These practices are made up of a limited number of patients (usually 500 to 600) and have a fixed annual membership fee ($1500 to $20,000).

Boutique practices usually provide these types of services:

1. The membership will cover what insurance does not, such as annual wellness exams
2. The time and attention to each patient as an individual and that quality care warrants
3. Your doctor is the only one you see unless he/she is out of town
4. Same-day appointment with a maximum 15-minute wait when needed
5. Each patient is seen for as long as they need and according to their need (an hour for a regularly scheduled annual check-up, half of an hour for other types of appointments)
6. Access to your physician 24/7 by having their email, fax, office, cell, and home numbers and they even will make house calls
7. Personal referral source and liaison for all medical care by other providers
8. A warm friendly staff who knows each patient as an individual
9. Beautifully decorated, comfortable offices with special amenities like beverages, fruit, other healthy snacks

There are lots of good reasons to become a member, but certainly these reasons help to reevaluate our medical care delivery system. Over the last 10 years, I have been following the growth and development of these boutique practices and, unfortunately, because of their attraction, some are gradually evolving into a semblance of our current group medical practices, just at a higher price.

Innovative Ideas for a Better US Healthcare Climate

Universal Health Care

First advocated by Germany's Otto von Bismarck in the 1880s, most German citizens are covered under a mandatory healthcare system. In 1948, the National Health Service (NHS) was established in the United Kingdom and is considered the world's first universal healthcare system provided by government that does include copays for certain procedures. In 1984, the Canada Health Act was passed and, for the most part, is publicly funded; physicians receive a fee per visit or service and are prohibited from extra billing. Most of the services are provided by private enterprises or private corporations, although most hospitals are public. Private pay services are available but carry financial disincentives unless the public system fails to deliver quality or timely service.

Retail Health Care

The United States has always been on the advanced and cutting edge of health care, from the Visiting Nurse Associations, which have all but completely been transformed into a plethora of home health agencies, to Medicare, the ground-breaking program for our elderly. Other very recent innovative healthcare delivery systems have not, as of yet, seen great success, such as physician and advanced practice nurse house call businesses like HouseCalls, MD AM/PM, Sick-day, and ACMI/900-ARNPNURSE. What has expanded quickly, but whose longevity has not been tested, are corporate-owned retail medical clinics, the most familiar being MinuteClinic. These retail healthcare clinics, staffed by medical and pediatric nurse practitioners who always collaborate with physicians and can practice independently in most states, are situated in pharmacy chains, grocery stores, and mass markets like Walmart, many of which have in-house pharmacies. The mission of these clinics is to provide sound medical care during regular business hours to relieve the excessive time and costs of unnecessarily using emergency rooms and provide quality care and savings without the long wait at the doctor's office for our millions of Medicaid, Medicare, underinsured, and uninsured citizens who become suddenly sick with common illnesses or sustain non–life-threatening injuries. Corporate America's modern revamping of home and emergency room visits could easily become an integral part of a truly unique comprehensive universal healthcare delivery system for the United States.

Under consideration by the US federal government since 1990, universal health care should not be confused with socialized medicine. The distinguishing characteristics of universal health care are:

1. Government action aimed at extending access to health care as widely as possible
2. Implemented through legislation and regulation which directs what care must be provided, to whom, and on what basis
3. Funded mostly or entirely by taxation, usually a combination of compulsory insurance and tax revenues with some costs assumed by the patient at the time of service
4. In some cases, government involvement also includes directly managing the healthcare system, but many countries use mixed public–private systems to deliver universal health care

The United States is the only wealthy, industrialized nation that does not have a universal healthcare system even though the government directly covers 27.8% of the population via Medicaid, Medicare, and other government subsidized welfare programs. According to a 2007 study by the Kaiser Family Foundation, since 2001 premiums for private family insurance coverage have increased 78% while inflation has risen 17% and wages have risen 19% (Palosky & Levitt, 2007). With statistics like this, the US government needs to address the cost, quality, and coverage for health care.

There have been numerous proposals to stimulate the current system into extending coverage more universally, rather than through a more comprehensive restructuring. Several studies have examined such market-based reform packages concluding that if market-oriented reforms are not implemented on a systematic basis with appropriate safeguards, they have the potential to cause more problems than they solve. Others have proposed that the whole US healthcare industry must be dismantled and built again from scratch. The author subscribes to a combination, with a heterogeneous team of knowledgeable people from various industries and professions who are both visionaries and strategic who can carefully plan and implement with conviction; can identify, admit, and shift quickly when something is not going correctly; and can rethink and implement again.

On November 5, 2008, President-elect Barack Obama promised to cut waste from the healthcare system and to introduce a universal healthcare plan into law by the end of his first term.

Our attention will next be on using nuggets of information about healthcare economics, identifying the challenges, and using critical and essential communication tools so we may join the wealthiest countries on the globe by creating a better and uniquely US healthcare climate: universal health care.

RECIPROCAL INFLUENCES ON HEALTH CARE

First kill all the lawyers.

—William Shakespeare

Managed care has not proven to be our healthcare delivery system panacea. US citizens are understandably confused about our overabundance of healthcare choices, which has lead to divided sentiment about "should we continue with our private payer systems or convert to a universal health care system?" National universal health care has been bandied about for more than 20 years. Fear of socialized medicine—understood by the general US population as a loss of choices—seems to be the greatest deterrent to the development of a universal healthcare system. Battista and McCabe (1999), researching the "American fear that universal health care would result in government control and intrusion into health care [would result] in loss of freedom of choice, [concluded that] single payer, universal health care administered by a state public health system would be much more democratic and much less intrusive than our current system. Consumers and providers [businesses and government] would have a voice in determining benefits, rates and taxes [resolving] problems with free choice, confidentiality and medical decision making." Battista and McCabe state that "single payer health care is not socialized medicine, any more than the public funding of education is socialized education, or the public funding of the defense industry is socialized defense." Battista and McCabe (1999) found that repeated national and state polls have shown that between 60 and 75% of Americans would like a universal healthcare system.

The United States spends 50 to 100% more on administration than single-payer systems in other countries. By lowering these administrative costs, the United States would have the ability to provide universal health care without managed care, with an increase in benefits, and still save money. Under a universal healthcare system all citizens could access care because there would be no lines, as in other industrialized countries, mainly because we have an oversupply in our providers and infrastructure and the willingness and ability of the United States to spend more on health care than other industrialized nations.

Now that we have a historical perspective, some interesting tidbits, and can conceptualize our complex and complicated healthcare delivery and practice systems, the following section will concentrate on the political, economic, and social reciprocal influences on our healthcare climate.

Politics

The United States is the only industrialized nation that does not guarantee access to health care as a right of citizenship. We continue to design healthcare delivery systems that support access based on the ability to pay, suggesting that health care is a privilege, often a privilege of the wealthy and the highly educated. Through lobbyists and the political donations allowed by our campaign finance system, corporations are able to buy politicians and control the media to convince people that corporate health care is democratic, represents freedom, and is the most efficient system for delivering health care.

Other than Germany, which has a multipayer universal healthcare system similar to the plan former President Clinton proposed for the United States in 1996, 28 industrialized nations have single-payer universal healthcare systems. The United States ranks poorly relative to other industrialized nations in health care despite having the best trained healthcare providers and the best medical infrastructure of any industrialized nation. Studies of state-administered healthcare plans by Massachusetts (universal health care was ratified and initiated there on July 1, 2007) and Connecticut (a notably "green" state studying single-payer universal health care) have shown that single-payer universal health care would save $1 to $2 billion per year from the total medical expenses in those states, despite covering all the uninsured and increasing healthcare benefits—due to lower administrative costs. Single-payer health care is not socialized medicine any more than the public funding of education is socialized education, or the public funding of the defense industry is socialized defense.

In the mid-20th century, rapid changes in our US healthcare and accounting systems were advanced by new politicians who were attorneys. This new legislative style led to an excess of amendments that resulted in layered-type changes, rather than substantive resolutions. Consequently, the government has played a greater role in making "ready-fire-aim" decisions for the healthcare industry. Halting the continuation of this political methodology is paramount to repairing our beleaguered healthcare system. Ready, aim, fire action means penetrating questions must come before answers and thoughtful and full analysis must precede planning.

A good start would be to consider these questions:

1. Why does the United States not have a single-payer universal healthcare system when it is apparent to most of the world that single-payer universal health care is the most efficient, most democratic, and most equitable means to deliver health care?
2. Why does the United States remain wedded to an inefficient, autocratic, easily abused healthcare delivery system that makes health care easily accessible to the wealthy and not the poor when a consistent majority of citizens want it to be a right of citizenship?
3. What would it really take for a democratic United States to redesign its antiquated, illness-oriented, corrupted, multipayer healthcare delivery system into a single-payer healthcare system that supports an efficient, fair, and equitable prevention-oriented system of "health" care?

Economics

Healthcare economics consists of a complicated relationship between a number of participants: the consumer, insurance companies, employers, medical professionals, and various government entities. An essential feature of healthcare economics is the spreading of risk, since the cost of health care for catastrophic illness can be prohibitive. This risk may be spread by private insurance companies who seek to make a profit or by government involvement in the healthcare market.

Understanding basic healthcare economics helps us in wisely choosing our personal healthcare insurer and providers, to support or oppose universal health care, and which active roles we might take in the political, business, and social healthcare arenas. The United States uses the gross domestic product (GDP), or what uses our money goes toward, as one benchmark for how the United States is doing economically. One study by global by consulting firm Price Waterhouse Coopers projected that global healthcare spending would triple in real dollars by 2020, consuming 21% of GDP in the United States and 16% of GDP in other Organization for Economic Cooperation and Development (OECD, a 30-member think tank) countries.

Funding models for healthcare delivery systems are extremely complex. Healthcare delivery systems can be funded by any number of models. In most countries with universal health care, funding has been achieved by a mixed model: private or public funds, or both, through a single- or multipayer system or state (municipal) and national funds provided through general taxation.

Risk compensation pools and compulsory insurance in free world economies are usually enforced by legislation that delineates whether one or several funds will provide basic services or extended services, or both. The economics of funding can include private or public and are used to equalize the risks between funds. Medicare is a risk compensation pool. A healthy, younger population pays into the fund and an older, predominantly less healthy population receives the funds. This type of pool competes on price so there is no advantage to eliminate people with higher risks because they are compensated for by means of risk-adjusted capitation payments. These types of funds are not allowed to pick and choose their policyholders or deny coverage, and the basic coverage level is set by the government and cannot be modified by individuals. Taxation in the United States sustains the public portion of healthcare insurance and may contribute, in part, to other forms of the private healthcare delivery system. This effectively meets the cost of insuring those unable to insure themselves via Social Security, as funded from taxation. Some countries, like the United Kingdom, Italy, and Spain, have eliminated insurance entirely and choose to fund health care directly from taxation. Other countries with insurance-based systems fund health care either by directly paying citizens' medical bills or by paying for insurance premiums for those affected.

Adverse selection, in simple terms, refers to those with poor health who are more likely to apply for insurance and more likely to need treatments requiring high insurance company payouts. Those with good health will often remove themselves from the risk pool, becoming the working uninsured, further raising costs. This gives private insurers an economic incentive to use medical underwriting to "weed out" high-cost applicants in order to avoid adverse selection. To avoid adverse selection and the continuous escalating costs of private healthcare insurance, economists offer, among the potential solutions, a single-payer system (see later discussion) ensuring that health insurance is universal, requiring all citizens to purchase insurance, and limiting the ability of insurance companies to deny insurance to individuals or vary price between individuals.

Single payer is the term used in the US debate over a universal healthcare system to describe the funding mechanism that would meet the costs of medical care from a single fund. Although the fund "holder" is assumed to be the government allocating funding from taxation to pay for health care, its proponents do not rule out the possibility of some other mechanism. It is therefore as of yet undetermined whether a future US single-payer universal healthcare system would be funded from taxation, from compulsory insurance, or a mixture of both. Many countries that have universal healthcare often provide private insurance as a supplement, as done in the United States with Medicare and Medicaid. Since the United States already has a functioning system in place, many of the universal healthcare proponents support adapting the existing system to create US universal health care. Private insurers might cover private rooms (United Kingdom), obtaining treatment more quickly than would otherwise be possible (Canada), or elective cosmetic surgery (Brazil).

From the beginning, the US healthcare delivery system was structured as free economy, multipayer organizations. Since 1970, the number of healthcare administrators has increased 23 times faster than the number of doctors and nurses. As of the early 1980s, the business of health care was taken out of the hands of physician administrators and private insurers (many of which were owned by individual or groups of physicians), and put into the hands of business people whose "ethics" are the bottom line. Since this transition, the ethics of practicing healthcare providers have come under harsh scrutiny. In single-payer universal health care everyone's health care would be paid for out of one publicly administered trust fund that would replace the current multipayer system, thereby eliminating the role of and need for insurance companies. It would provide all residents with comprehensive healthcare coverage that assures the freedom to choose physicians, nurse practitioners, and other healthcare professionals, services, and facilities.

True or False?

The United States has the best healthcare system in the world. Universal health care would be too expensive. Universal health care would deprive citizens of needed services. The problems with the US healthcare system are being solved and are best solved by private, corporate, managed care medicine because they are the most efficient. Battista and McCabe (1999) conclude that these statements are all false by citing the following:

- The United States ranks 23rd in infant mortality, down from 12th in 1960 and 21st in 1990.
- The United States ranks 20th in life expectancy for women, down from 1st in 1945 and 13th in 1960.
- The United States ranks 21st in life expectancy for men, down from 1st in 1945 and 17th in 1960.
- The United States ranks between 50th and 100th in immunizations, depending on the immunization. Overall the United States is 67th, right behind Botswana.
- Outcome studies on a variety of diseases, such as coronary artery disease and renal failure, show the United States to rank below Canada and a wide variety of industrialized nations.
- The United States ranks poorly relative to other industrialized nations in health care despite having the best trained healthcare providers and the best medical infrastructure of any industrialized nation.
- For-profit, managed care cannot solve the US healthcare problems because health care is not a commodity that people shop for and the quality of care will always be compromised when the motivating factor for corporations is to save money through denial of care and decreasing provider costs.
- Managed care has introduced problems of patient confidentiality and disrupted the continuity of care by having limited provider networks.
- Private, for-profit corporations are the least efficient deliverer of health care. They spend between 20 and 30% of premiums on administration and profits. The public sector is the most efficient. Medicare spends 3% on administration.
- The same procedure in the same hospital, the year after conversion from not-for-profit to for-profit, costs between 20 and 35% more.
- Healthcare costs in the United States grew more under managed care in 1990 to 1996 than any other industrialized nation with single-payer universal health care.
- Since the late 1980s, the quality of health care in the United States has deteriorated under managed care. Access problems have increased and the number of uninsured has dramatically increased—10 million to 43.4 million from 1989 to 1995, 16% in 1996, and increasing each year.
- The level of satisfaction with the US healthcare system is the lowest of any industrialized nation. Eighty percent of US citizens and 71% of US doctors believe that managed care has caused quality of care to be compromised.

According to a 2007 World Health Organization (WHO) report, the United States had the most expensive health care of any OECD country and also had the highest percentage of costs paid privately, with some of the worst health statistics in the free world.

Social

The social facet of our influence is determined by the arena of our target audience. The social aspect of professional healthcare practice refers to our patients and clients, colleagues, students, meetings we attend and present at, locations in which we function professionally, and the professional organizations we actively join. The social part of politics concerns our local and regional state offices and officers, state and national legislators, our President and his executives, our national centers and committees, and the organizations and committees in which we are publically active and about which we speak. The social side of economics is about our relationships with our bankers, investment counselors, financiers, and our state and national legislators and the committees on which they serve. We share our interactions in our social life with our families, friends, and acquaintances at sporting events, parties, and gatherings. Professional practice, politics, economics, and society are intertwined and related to the topic of healthcare reform. It is in the socializing setting of each area that the tools we use to communicate with our target audience matter the most.

In our healthcare practices, we use all the technology and electronic tools at hand: email, fax, phone, Internet information, blogs, and social internet sites; networking; written material for professional journals and books; general interest magazines and books; teaching; photography; and professional and public speaking engagements. In addition to these same contact tools, when in the political and economic fields, we use our verbal assets and face-to-face meetings to their utmost such as networking, educating, lobbying, campaigning, assistance in writing legislation (new amendments, referenda), and participating in activities and meetings. In our social and family circles we count mostly on social gatherings, networking (personal and technological), and informed, hopefully passionate, discussion.

THE FUTURE OF US HEALTH CARE

Future Challenges

The US healthcare system has three primary goals: the provision of high quality care, ready access to the system, and affordable costs. Certain causes of healthcare inflation are desirable and inevitable, such as the development of new drugs and technologies and an aging population. However, other causes of soaring healthcare costs are clearly less defensible. These include the high administrative costs of the US healthcare system, our litigious culture that results in the high price of defensive medicine, a profligate US practice style in which many doctors often perform unnecessary tests and procedures, the inflationary consequences of having a third party pay the bill (thereby removing incentives from both doctors and patients to conserve dollars), and the existence of for-profit managed care organizations and hospital chains that each year divert billions of dollars of healthcare premiums away from medical care and into private wealth. Clearly, there is much room to operate a more efficient, responsible healthcare delivery system in the United States at a more affordable price.

Today's Issues and Trends Facing US Health Care

Efficient Use of Resources

The wiser and more efficient use of resources is only one challenge to the US healthcare system. In this 21st century, the United States will still face the problem of limited resources and seemingly limitless demand. At some point hard decisions will have to be made about what services will and will not be paid for. Any efforts at cost containment must continue to be balanced with efforts to maintain high quality and patient advocacy in medical care. Better access to the system must also be provided. The US public must maintain realistic expectations of medicine. This can be done by recognizing broad determinants of health like good education and meaningful employment, avoiding the *medicalization* of social ills like crime and drug addiction, and recognizing that individuals must assume responsibility for their own health by choosing a healthy lifestyle. Only when all of these issues are satisfactorily taken into account will the US have a healthcare delivery system that matches the promise of what medical science and practice have to offer.

Fraud, Abuse, and Waste

The multipayer US healthcare system, which is so complex, multilayered, confusing, conflicting, and overrun with unceasing paperwork, provides fertile ground for fraud, abuse, and waste that runs unchecked. A single-payer universal healthcare system by definition could provide the checks and balances missing in the existing healthcare delivery system.

The Joint Commission Monopoly

The Joint Commission is akin to what would be a single-payer healthcare system in that it holds the monopoly on accreditation of hospitals for Medicare. In this case, hospital accreditation among competitive agencies could strengthen standards and streamline the very difficult and anxiety-provoking process of accreditation.

Rural Medicine

In rural areas there is and will continue to be a physician shortage. Medical insurance alone will not solve the health problems of a poor rural community where there are no hospitals, doctors, clinics, or pharmacies. Public health systems and an array of alternative primary care providers often fill in the gaps. Primary care may be provided by nurse practitioners, physician assistants, or home-health nurses. Practice locations include publicly or charitably subsidized comprehensive primary care centers, specialty service clinics, and in patient homes. Advances in medical technology, increasing costs, and market forces contribute to the economic destabilization of many rural healthcare systems and the closings of hospitals. Consequently, rural residents must often travel great distances to access more costly and complex levels of care.

Aging Population

Neither Medicare nor the National Agency on Aging provides plans of care for the elderly. Life expectancy and the quality and costs of care in the United States, and around the globe, are increasing without plans to care for and house the aging population. An opportunity exists for the United States to provide innovative initiatives and cost planning for health care and housing communities for the aging in its healthcare reform.

Healthcare Provider Shortages

A shortage of physicians and advanced practice nurses, an increase in the relatively new positions of physician assistant and nursing technician, and an increase of pharmacists are expected in 2010. Many physicians and nurse practitioners have left health care for the business world and creative endeavors, therefore purging inspired, brilliant, and talented people from health care. Medical providers have seen managed care companies and executives of healthcare businesses making much more money than healthcare providers who save lives every day. Some healthcare providers feel invalidated and devalued by the predominant managed care companies. Others believe that the managed care mindset and lack of sensitivity and professional ethics have almost eradicated the art of the science and practice of health care. Because most physicians, advanced practice nurses, and patients believe that universal health care and a single-payer system will improve practice conditions for providers and quality of care for patients, US residents must become actively involved in healthcare reform.

Controlling Costs

As costs increase, public and private insurers must struggle to control their expenditures. In the 2009 recession, subscribers are also controlling expenditures—many, unfortunately, are doing so by cutting back on doctor visits and not following or filling prescriptions. Many believe that universal health care with a single-payer system is the answer. Until this hotly debated issue can be settled, cost containment will remain the primary problem of the multipayer healthcare delivery system.

Resurrecting the Healthcare System: The Next Step

The United States has the most expensive health care in the world. US citizens have become a population used to high-priced, over marketed and advertised designer medications and the most current and expensive diagnostic and treatment technology. The present over-65 Medicare population believed that it could well afford these medications and treatments before an economic recession began in earnest in 2007, depositing the United States firmly in the worst economic climate ever recorded. Citizens and government officials overwhelmingly agree that the US system, the most expensive health care system in the world, is broken; I venture that it is irreparably broken and the only solution is a universal healthcare, single-payer system.

A universal healthcare single-payer system appears to be the only solution to saving the future of the US healthcare system. Economic concerns about the constantly escalating costs of healthcare services, scientific research and development, the manufacturing of medical technologies and designer drugs; national worries about a severe economic recession; popular citizen opinion; and support by the healthcare provider community and President Obama make this the second most important agenda item, warranting a solution by the Obama administration. Unless the universal health care dispute is settled in a positive direction, the United States will continue to be plagued by the aforementioned concerns. The following pros and cons highlight the current universal healthcare and single-payer system debate.

Common arguments by supporters of universal healthcare systems include:

- Ensuring the health of all citizens benefits a nation economically.
- A single-payer system could save $286 billion a year in overhead and paperwork. One estimate put the total administrative costs at 24% of US healthcare spending.
- Wastefulness and inefficiency in the delivery of health care would be reduced.
- The United States spends a far higher percentage of GDP on health care than any other country but has worse ratings on such criteria as quality of care, efficiency of care, access to care, safe care, equity, and wait times, according to the Commonwealth Fund (foundation established 1918 by Anna M. Harkness, "for the welfare of mankind").
- The profit motive adversely affects the cost and quality of health care.
- Universal health care and public doctors would protect the right to privacy between insurance companies and patients.

Common arguments by opponents of universal healthcare systems include:

- Health care is not a right; as such, it is not the responsibility of government to provide health care.
- Unequal access and health disparities still exist in universal healthcare systems.
- The widely quoted healthcare system ranking by WHO, in which the US system ranked below other countries' universal healthcare systems, used biased criteria, giving a false sense of those systems' superiority.
- Large market-based public programs such as the Federal Employees Health Benefits Program can provide better coverage than Medicare while still controlling costs as well.

COMMUNICATION AND THE PRESENT HEALTHCARE CLIMATE

I am not a teacher, but an awakener.

—Robert Frost

Business would be great if it weren't for the people.

—Anonymous

Communication and Change

Like the importance of history as a communicator of information about our past accomplishments and mistakes, some psychological history about human communication would be valuable here. For all of our intellectual gifts and verbal abilities, human beings continuously get caught on the spikes of childhood experiences; cultural, religious, and family teachings; personal situations; and emotional encounters that leave us with fears of criticism and rejection—fears of loss of esteem, position, money. People are resilient and courageous. We make mistakes and do our best to learn and communicate our shortcomings, ideas, wishes, needs, wants, and even our assets with the hope of not seeming egotistical.

But change is not easy for us. Some of us welcome and embrace change as the challenge that it is; however, most of us are change averse. Driven by our unconscious, we perceive change as loss in that we have to give up something to gain something else, and the devil we know will always be more comfortable to live with than the devil we do not know. Loss is the bottom-line issue for people; facing the ultimate loss: our own mortality. Change can only happen if we raise our awareness of our motivations, learn from our feelings and actions, and use all the available tools of communication. New learning happens only by careful and strategic examination of our mistakes and accomplishments, curious looks at past motivations and behaviors, analysis of the information, and development of a strategic plan for change. Implementation is the weakest point of any plan, and implementation is communication.

The Communication Imperative

When planning healthcare change, using communication as an imperative creates a whole new culture by raising strategic planning standards and generating decisive actions. Healthcare providers have always embraced change as a challenge to grow, and communication as a teacher and informant for enhanced learning and performance. If we are to change our healthcare system and climate, we must learn to communicate more skillfully with each other. We are graced with an overabundance of tools of communication, both verbal and nonverbal. The first part of great communication is recognizing that there are no dumb questions and that asking is often more important than getting answers. The second part of great communication is functioning successfully in a group or on a team. The third part is the greater communication skill: listening. We listen with all of our senses. Constructive, goal-oriented communication is the sharing of ideas, opinions, thoughts, impressions, and feelings. Attentive, active listening and observing will often provide more information than actively engaging in passionately heated conversation. Asking, "Do we want to reform, remodel, or rebuild our healthcare delivery system?" provides infinitely more success than struggling over the pros and cons of universal health care and a single-payer system. Discussing whether health care is a right or a privilege is more wasteful of communication energy and time than asking, "How do other countries succeed at having a universal healthcare system that provides both for their citizens?" What we may discover is that we need to think about a system that values fair and equitable versus one that values fair and equal. Is it acceptable for all residents to receive levels of good and more than adequate health care in a financially solvent climate, instead of adequate or excellent care in a financially bankrupt one? Do our principles of free enterprise in our democratically run country conflict with a universal healthcare and single-payer system? Starting with these and other realistic communiqués is the place to begin when designing a fresh and viable healthcare delivery system, be it a universal single-payer or a private multipayer solution.

JOURNALING EXERCISES

1. History Exercise

You are taking a class on History of American Health Care at the local university that began 2 weeks ago. Your professor walks into class last night quoting Konrad Adenauer (chancellor of Federal Republic of Germany, 1949 to 1963, who must rank as the most successful German politician since 1945): "History is the sum total of the things that could have been avoided." Your professor assigns the class to keep a journal this semester. Record responses to questions like:

What does the quote say to you?

What have we learned from healthcare history that should have been avoided?

Why, for we humans, does history repeats itself so often?

What can we do about avoiding history repeating itself?

What does US healthcare history teach us that we need to remain cognizant of so as not to repeat the same mistakes when the US government gets around to designing a universal, single-payer healthcare system?

_____

_____

_____

_____

_____

_____

_____

_____

2. The Business of Health Care

What are six characteristics that make the US healthcare system and healthcare climate unique?

How do they make the US healthcare delivery system and healthcare climate unique?

_____

_____

_____

_____

_____

_____

_____

_____

3. Navigating Medicare and Medicaid

Your 20-year-old patient on dialysis and her mother have a first appointment with you in 2 days. As with all first complex appointments, you schedule them for a 40-minute visit with 20 minutes of after time for you to make additional notes in your sourcing journal. This family was referred to you because of your in-depth knowledge about the practices and practicalities of healthcare delivery systems, and your ability to communicate this to patients is legendary in the healthcare community. As this family is new to permanent disability, they require your help in navigating the appropriate systems and maximizing their benefits. You spend 15 minutes creating a patient sourcing journal outline that includes, but is not limited to, the following:

What the family needs to know about:

- Medicaid is their primary insurer and Medicare is the supplemental insurer when the patient is on permanent disability (SSI)
- Filling out the required Medicaid and Medicare forms
- What benefits Medicaid will and will not cover
- What supplemental benefits Medicare covers
- Your ethical guidelines about billing practices
- How you conduct your practice
- The advantages and limits of your credentials and practice
- Your availability during and after office hours

Sideline notes are added according to the needs of the patient and family regarding:

- Your and their communication styles
- Your and their surfacing feelings
- The amount of information that they can absorb, in what time period
- Your impressions of their comprehension levels

- Assessment of all aspects of their levels of functioning
- Assessment of their physical, emotional, social, and financial resources

What are the similarities and differences between managed care reform of the late 20th century and universal healthcare reform of the early 21st century? Take your time and compile a list. Share the list with your legislators and medical associations and the local newspaper and radio talk show program. Write a book.

_____

_____

_____

_____

_____

_____

_____

4. Healthcare Systems

Because of your many recognition awards for superior public speaking skills and commendations for innovative medical practice, you have been asked by your alma mater to deliver this year's 20-minute graduation address. The dean requested that you speak on (surprise, surprise) innovative healthcare models. You came up with a sexy title, "Universal and retail health care: Strange bedfellows." In planning out the speech, you developed several headings:

What are they?

What do universal and retail health care have in common?

How do they differ?

Explain how retail health care be an integral part of a universal healthcare system.

Fill in the blanks and you have a speech.

_____

_____

_____

_____

_____

_____

_____

_____

5. Politics and Communication Imperatives

Because of your known interest in becoming actively involved in the politics and legislative process of health care and healthcare reform, you have been invited to participate with a team of healthcare professionals to develop and bring a healthcare reform referendum to the state legislature. Now is your golden opportunity. Having never done this before, you want to go in somewhat prepared so no one will think you are a complete novice. So you ask two other advanced practice colleagues to come over to your house on Wednesday night for 2 hours of drinks (nothing too strong), nibbles (nothing too fattening), and role play for the practice and experience of what it might actually be like to do the job requested of you. You chose John and Marie because they will challenge you and even throw in a little intimidation for the experience—John not too much the expert and Marie not exactly a novice. Lots are drawn for who you each will be impersonating. Marie is the lobbyist with 4 years of experience under her belt. John is the old-school legislative whip with womanizing tendencies—you heard from a very reliable source that, 15 years ago, he salaciously asked an advanced practice registered nurse (APRN) lobbyist what she would do for him if he sponsored her bill and she replied "Not report you" (a tough act to follow!). You are the team's newbie healthcare member and their spokesperson who will be presenting the referendum to the lobbyist and legislator together.

What feelings do you have when initially thinking about this opportunity?

How do you feel about the new dual role as member and spokesperson? How will you approach your role as newest team member? And team spokesperson?

What behaviors do you anticipate will be exhibited toward you as the newbie by the other team members? What might be motivating their behaviors?

What communication tools do you anticipate using at your first team meeting?

What verbal and nonverbal communications are the team members using?

During the role play, how will you communicate with John and Marie about what you need from them to make this role play realistic?

What feelings do you think the role play will bring out about the referendum presentation meeting?

What work will you need to do on your more objectionable feelings? On strengthening your strong points?

What communication tools can you anticipate using when dealing with the lobbyist and legislator?

How will you communicate strength and influence with these political powerbrokers?

What information do you need to have to present an effective, persuasive referendum?

_____

_____

_____

_____

_____

_____

_____

_____

6. Cost Containment in Health Care

The15 leading causes of death in the United States in 2007 fell into these Seven *International Statistical Classification of Diseases, 10th revision* (ICD-10) diagnostic categories:

1. Diseases of heart (heart disease)
2. Malignant neoplasms (cancer)
3. Cerebrovascular diseases (stroke)
4. Chronic lower respiratory diseases
5. Accidents (unintentional injuries)
6. Diabetes mellitus (diabetes)
7. Alzheimer's disease

Develop a four-module program to educate the public on preventative care and current treatments regarding these disease entities.

Design a simple, cost-effective marketing and advertising campaign and tools to let the public know what the program is, who is teaching it, where it will be held, on what days, what times will it be offered, who the sponsor is (can be for name recognition or funding), and what is the consumer's cost for the program—donate the cost to a medical charity, it is tax deductible and does a lot of good.

Include these aspects of prevention in this program:

- Document that prevention is more cost effective than treatment.
- Teach the steps of preventative medicine that improves health and reduces disease.
- List five signs with which patients can identify each disease process.
- Identify and describe the current treatments for these diseases.
- In what ways do informed and educated healthcare consumers contribute to containment of healthcare costs?

You will need your personal teaching tools and the following supplies at each meeting:

- Good lighting and enough comfortable classroom style seating that preferably can be converted into auditorium and circle seating
- Pads of paper and pens, some colored
- Good drinking water, ice, cups, and trash bags
- Hard sucking candies, some sugar free
- Fruit, napkins, plastic ware, small paper plates
- Anything else you want

_____

_____

_____

_____

_____

_____

_____

7. Social Influence

Talk to two coworkers, friends, and family members as separate pairs about why single-payer finance and universal healthcare legislation will improve quality, access, and affordability of care. The following are reform issues to be considered during the discussion:

Reduced spending versus reduced utilization

Reduced spending versus raising taxes

Reduced services versus increased beneficiary contributions

Increased services versus increased out of pocket expenditures

Managed care versus universal health care

Fee for services versus access to care

Age eligibility versus benefit income ceiling

Take as long as you want to discuss. Have a third person be a recorder. Compile and organize the data in three concept areas: improving quality, access, and affordability of care. Write a report and submit it for acceptance at a healthcare conference of your choice. Do not give up if rejected by the first conference committee. Remember, if you throw enough, some of it will stick.

_____

_____

_____

_____

_____

_____

_____

_____

8. Future Challenges

What are the US medical industry's healthcare challenges regarding:

- High administration costs?
- An aging culture and citizenry?
- Defensive medicine to combat a litigious society?
- Continuing numbers of unnecessary tests and procedures?

- Inflationary consequences of third-party payers?
- For-profit managed care?

_____

_____

_____

_____

_____

_____

_____

9. Trends and Issues

Write a succinct one-page letter to your local newspaper urging support of creating a single-payer universal healthcare system in your state. Feel free to cite the successes of Kaiser-Permanente, Massachusetts, Connecticut, Maryland, and California.

Make your points clearly and succinctly because long sentences and long letters are not read or printed unless they are very seductive or controversial.

Name four of the top trends and issues plaguing our present multipayer managed care healthcare delivery systems.

List two describers each for the up and down sides of the four trends and issues you named.

End by concisely stating the case for the healthcare system that you believe will reform and save our flagging healthcare system.

Sign your name and list and fully spell out the names of your credentials with the parenthetical acronym after each credential. Send the letter.

_____

_____

_____

_____

_____

_____

_____

_____

10. Single-Payer Universal Healthcare System

Your department chair has started a study group that meets at her home on Wednesday nights, 7–9 PM. This is the reading list:

1. *The Corrosion of Medicine: Can the Profession Reclaim Its Moral Legacy?* by John Geyman, MD.
2. Publications on healthcare reform by the Massachusetts Nurses Association.
3. Any number of books by Marcia Angell, MD (a past president of the Massachusetts Medical Association and former editor of *The New England Journal of Medicine*).
4. Healthcare books published by Common Courage Press, Monroe, Maine.

She said that these are important publications written by seasoned, experienced physicians and healthcare professionals and they address the ills of the present healthcare system and encourage launching new healthcare reform by supporting a universal healthcare single-payer system.

The topic of the study group for the next 6 weeks is staying current on the issues and questions regarding single-payer universal healthcare as it affects your organization, patients, third-party payers, and the practice of health care.

Participants have been asked to keep a journal of their response to the issues raised and solutions provided and to come to study group prepared to share and discuss them. Twenty to 30 minutes of journaling time per 2 hours of reading is recommended (more if you want), to be divided among the following:

Reactions
Feelings
Thoughts
Questions
Objections
Support
Insights
Other issues
Your solutions

---

11. Communication and Change

Friends, family, and colleagues have been bombarding you for years, and more so lately, about running for city office. You are finally weakening, it has been something you have always entertained ever since you can remember. You go to city hall and declare your candidacy for city council member. You have assembled your political strategy committee and it is time to plan and implement a strategy. These are some of the questions that have been raised that need answers to develop your campaign. Your committee wants you to flesh out your ideas and answers by the next meeting in 3 days. Successfully communicating your plans for change are paramount to winning the city council seat.

Why do you want to run?

Whose help do you need to wage a successful run, and why do you need them?

Who is your constituency, your target audience, who do you need to reach?

What platform would you run on regarding these areas and their issues?

> Health care
> Education
> Politics
> Economics
> Business
> Social issues
> Safety

What communication tools do you want to use to convey your platform and ideas for change?

_____

_____

_____

_____

_____

12. Corporate Culture

Dr. Madeleine Leininger, distinguished nursing researcher and theoretician, recognized for contributing the *cultural diversity and universality theory* to the practice of nursing, has been invited to your hospital to speak to advanced practice clinicians for 1 hour, followed by 40 minutes of coffee and discussion. At the heart of her theory is the "emphasis on the importance of cultural knowledge and of shaping care practices to be culturally congruent and applicable beyond nursing practice [and] can be used in a wide variety of situations" and disciplines (George, 2002, p. 578). You are very excited about attending because you recently started seriously reading about the importance of organizational culture learning and learned that each healthcare delivery system in our multipayer healthcare system has a different corporate culture which informs its ways of communicating that affects the total US healthcare climate. To prepare to get the most out of this lecture you think about and answer these questions yourself; you hope very much to also ask Dr. Leininger some of them.

How would I define my organization's corporate culture?

How would I describe the effects our corporate culture has on the healthcare climate at our organization? On our patients and their families?

How do the different payers' cultures affect the way we do business?

What effect does my hospital's culture have on the way we deliver health care?

How does my organization's culture affect its own healthcare climate and that of the United States?

What are the differences and similarities between my organization's culture and the multipayers' cultures?

In what ways does my organization effectively communicate?

In what ways does my organization communication ineffectively?

In what ways are corporate cultures and communication systems separate yet interdependent variables?

_____

_____

_____

_____

_____

_____

_____

_____

REFERENCES

Battista, J. R., & McCabe, J. (1999). *The case for single payer, universal health care for the United States.* Speech at the Connecticut Coalition for Universal Health Care, Moodus, CT.

Benner, P. (1984). *From novice to expert: excellence and power in clinical nursing practice.* Menlo Park, CA: Addison-Wesley.

Buber, M. (1970). *I and thou* (W. Kaufmann, Trans.). New York: Charles Scribner Sons. (Original work published 1937)

Buckman, E. S. (1994). *Handbook of humor: Clinical applications in psychotherapy.* Malabar, FL: Krieger.

Dreyfus, H. L., & Dreyfus, S. E. (1986). *Mind over machine: The power of human intuition and expertise in the age of the computer.* Oxford: Basil Blackwell.

George, J., (Ed.). (2002). *Nursing theories: The base for professional practice* (5th ed.). Upper Saddle River, NJ: Prentice Hall.

Kung, H. C., Hoyert, D. L., Xu, J. Q., & Murphy, S. L. (2008). *Deaths: Final data for 2005 for National Vital Statistics Reports.* (Vol. 56, no. 10). Hyattsville, MD: U.S. Department of Health and Human Services, Centers for Disease Control and Prevention, National Center for Health Statistics. Publication CS117176 T31006 (04/2008), DHHS Publication No. (PHS) 2008-1120.

Orlando, I. J. (1961). *The dynamic nurse-patient relationship, function, process and principles.* New York: G. P. Putnam.

Palosky, C., & Levitt, L. (2007, September 11). 2007 Kaiser/HRET employer health benefits survey. Retrieved May 13, 2009, from http://www.kff.org/insurance/ehbs091107nr.cfm

Peplau, H. (1952). *Interpersonal relations in nursing.* New York: Springer Publishing Co.

Ridgway, C. (2008). Evaluating the Obama-Biden health care plan. *Convenient Care, 3*(1), 10.

Rogers, C. R. (1951). *Client-centered therapy.* Boston: Houghton Mifflin.

Sullivan, H. S. (1953). *The interpersonal theory of psychiatry.* New York: W. W. Norton.

Temkin, O., & Temkin, C. L. (1967). Ancient medicine: selected papers of Ludwig Edelstein. In O. Temkin & C. L. Temkin (Eds.), *The Hippocratic oath: Text, translation and interpretation.* Baltimore: Johns Hopkins Press.

SUGGESTED READINGS

Arnett, R. C. (1986). *Communication and community: Implications of Martin Buber's dialogue.* Carbondale, IL: Southern Illinois University Press.

Birenbaum, A. (1997). *Managed care: Made in America.* Westport, CT: Praeger.

Centers for Medicare and Medicaid Services, U.S. Department of Health and Human Services. (n.d.). Retrieved May 13, 2009, from http://www.cms.hhs.gov

Committee on Consequences of Uninsurance of the Institute of Medicine at the National Academies of Science. (2004). *Insuring America's health: principles and recommendations.* Washington, DC: National Academies Press.

Dranove, D. (2000). *The economic evolution of American health care: From Marcus Welby to managed care.* Princeton, NJ: Princeton University Press.

Dreyfus, H. L., & Dreyfus, S. E. (1996). Expertise in nursing practice: Caring, clinical judgment, and ethics. In P. Benner, C. Tanner, & C. Chesla (Eds.), *The relationship of theory and practice in the acquisition of skill* (pp. 29–40). New York: Springer Publishing Co.

Erikson, E. (1963). *Childhood and society.* New York: W. W. Norton and Co.

Frankl, V. E. (1984). *Man's search for meaning* (3rd ed.). New York: Simon & Schuster, Inc.

Fuchs, V. R. (1986). *The health economy.* Cambridge, MA: Harvard University Press.

Gray, B. H. (1991). *The profit motive and patient care: The changing accountability of doctors and hospitals.* Cambridge, MA: Harvard University Press.

Lundberg, G. D. (2000). *Severed trust: Why American medicine hasn't been fixed.* New York: Basic Books.

Maslow, A. (1970). *Motivation and personality* (2nd ed.). New York: Harper and Row.

Neuman, B., & Fawcett, J. (Eds.). (2002). *The Neuman systems model* (4th ed.). Upper Saddle River, NJ: Prentice Hall.

Oberlander, J. (2003). *Political life of Medicare.* Chicago: University of Chicago Press.

Parker, M. E., (Ed.). (2001). *Nursing theories and nursing practice.* Philadelphia: F.A. Davis Co.

Robbins, D. (1998). *Managed care on trial: Recapturing trust, integrity, and accountability in healthcare.* New York: McGraw-Hill.

Rogers, C. R. (1942). *Counseling and psychotherapy.* Boston: Houghton Mifflin.

Schein, E. J. (1988). *Process consultation revisited: Building the helping relationship* (2nd ed.). Reading, MA: Addison-Wesley.

Schein, E. J. (1998). *Process consultation: It's role in organizational development.* Reading, MA: Addison-Wesley.

Selye, H. (1950). *The physiology and pathology of exposure to stress.* Montreal, Quebec, Canada: Acta, Inc.

Tomey, A. M., & Alligood, M. R., (Eds.). (2002). *Nursing theorists and their work* (5th ed.). St Louis, MO: Mosby.

Von Bertalanffy, L. (1968). *General systems theory.* New York: Braziller.

CHAPTER 3

Personal and Professional Relationships and Communication

Valerie A. Hart

One of the most complex concepts in the area of role development is the professional versus the personal role when dealing with patients. It is a difficult concept because it requires the capacity of both connection and detachment, and erring on either dimension will cause major problems for the provider–patient relationship. Beginning clinicians are often confused about what constitutes connection, either in the words they use or the physical acts of connection, such as a touch of the hand or giving a patient a hug. They may also be as confused about what is the appropriate level of disengagement or detachment in the professional role. How does one avoid being flooded emotionally by the difficult realities of terminal cancer, chronic illness, or death? How does one convey a sense of caring while maintaining the ability to separate at the end of the clinical encounter and enter into another experience with another patient? How does one protect oneself from the stress of emotional wear-and-tear of the work so that burnout or compassion fatigue does not occur? How does the clinician retain a reservoir of empathy that may be needed at the end of day for one's family members? All of these questions are vitally important to understand and problem solve in order to create and sustain a satisfying professional practice that can endure over time.

Over the years, I have had many conversations with graduate students, often nurses with many years of experience, in the area of sharing personal information and self-disclosure. What is okay to share, and how personal can one be? Is it helpful or detrimental to the nurse–patient relationship to do so? How does one begin a therapeutic relationship without first sharing on a personal level? How do I handle when a patient is too curious about me or my family? What tools assist me when either I or the patient has crossed a boundary in this relationship?

It has been shown that when clinicians *perceive* patients to be like them they are able to experience empathetic engagement, yet a patient's familiarity with the clinician is *not* an important factor in their engaging with them (Makoul & Strauss, 2003).

BOUNDARIES

Professional boundaries are the framework parameters within which health care is delivered. Regardless of how egalitarian the healthcare provider wishes to be, there is an inherent power differential when treating patients. This is because one person is providing care and the other is paying a fee for those services. Boundaries are rules of behavior and are a way to describe the limits of the professional relationship. Boundaries that are clear to both providers and patients provide a safe environment within which to provide care. Boundary issues include issues of self-disclosure, length of clinical visits, the use of touch, and the overall manner of relating to the patient. Boundary issues also include keeping secrets with patients, accepting gifts, and altering one's dress when caring for a patient. While patients and families may push at boundaries, it is the clinician who generally establishes the parameters. Managing boundary issues is a component of professional practice, along with the mandate to act in the patient's best interest at all times. Along with self-disclosure, which will be discussed at length, other areas that relate to boundaries are situations of overlapping roles and the question of making friends with a patient. In the former situation, the clinician may find themselves involved with a patient on a social or personal level, such as serving on a committee at one's church, treating a patient who is in a class with you, or is your child's teacher. These situations blur boundaries between personal and professional functioning and are tricky to navigate. In a similar vein, attempting to balance having friendships with patients/clients can be confusing, even if tempting. Giving a patient special attention or treatment, unlike other patients under your care, may be a warning sign for a potential violation of boundaries. Inviting a patient to a dinner party you are having, asking a patient to help you move or to paint your new apartment, and asking a patient to see a movie with you are all examples of crossing boundaries.

Inappropriate familiarity when addressing a patient or referring to the patient by use of their first name or nickname rather than beginning with a more formal address can be seen as a boundary issues. A clinician needs to know the patient's preference in terms of how they would like to be addressed; asking the patient directly is the easiest approach, as it is never wise to assume what this preference might be.

The issue of physical contact in a professional encounter needs to be negotiated, not assumed. Beyond a professional handshake, physical touch that is uninvited, such as a hug, can be misunderstood and make patients feel unsafe. It is advisable to ask a patient if physical contact is alright, which allows the patient to communicate their preferences in this area.

Discussions about boundaries aimed at the lay population are quite common in literature focused on sexual abuse. For example, The Treehouse offers guidelines for examining whether provider behavior is appropriate or has crossed boundaries (Treehouse, 2006). Providers can ask themselves a series of questions about potential boundary violations (Box 3-1):

The ultimate boundary violation in a patient–provider relationship is that of sexual contact. Most healthcare disciplines have clear prohibitions in regard to this behavior, and there are also legal and ethical constraints to consider. There is no situation that permits sexual contact between patient and provider. It is the most serious breach of trust in a therapeutic relationship that can occur. The literature on this topic often discusses warning signs that a clinician may have when treating a client, including feeling sexually drawn to them or sharing highly personal information with a patient, but it may also include fantasizing or dreaming about sexual encounters with a patient. These warning signs ought to inform the provider that they need to discuss these thoughts

Box 3-1   Nursing Education Models

Is this in my client's best interest?
Whose needs are being served?
Will this have an impact on the service I am delivering?
Should I make a note of my concerns or consult with a colleague?
How would this be viewed by the client's family or significant other?
How would I feel telling a colleague about this?
Am I treating this client differently (e.g., appointment length, time of appointments, extent of personal disclosures)?
Does this client mean something special to me?
Am I taking advantage of the client?
Does this action benefit me rather than the client?
Am I comfortable in documenting this decision/behavior in the client file?
Does this contravene regulations, written Standards of Professional Conduct, or the Code of Ethics for the certifying group I belong to, etc.?

and feelings with a colleague or supervisor, or in a peer group. It is not the countertransference itself that is dangerous. The danger lies in refusing to acknowledge the thoughts and feelings. Denial of these may lead to acting them out with a patient. Providers need to be alert to their own behavior and take note if their behavior toward patients has a sexual tone. Slips of the tongue are windows to the unconscious and, if sexual in nature, may warn the clinician to engage in self-reflection.

SELF-DISCLOSURE

Provider self-disclosure involves sharing personal information with patients, as well as aspects of the self that are not obvious such as feelings, thoughts, or attitudes (Servellen, 2009). Zur (2008) classifies self-disclosures as:

Deliberate
Unavoidable
Accidental
As a result of client action

Deliberate self-disclosure includes any intentional sharing of personal information by a clinician. This may include both verbal and nonverbal sharing. The latter might include displaying personal items in one's office, including family photos or a child's artwork. In this category the clinician makes a conscious choice to either reveal or not hide personal information from patients. Sharing how one spends personal time, hobbies one engages in, or where an upcoming vacation destination is are examples of deliberate self-disclosure.

Unavoidable self-disclosure involves the realities of who the clinician is, such as gender and age as well as issues such as pregnancy, obesity, style of dress, office décor taste, and the presence of an injury or disability. If the clinician is using a cane, or has an ankle wrapped in a compression bandage, it reveals aspects of their life that may not be otherwise part of the patient–provider conversation.

Accidental self-disclosure is just that. Getting out of one's car in the parking lot of the practice site might reveal the type of car a clinician drives, and bumping into a clinician at a social event or a restaurant or the mall may introduce the patient to the patient's family or significant other. Any of these situations may reveal economic status of the clinician, or at least begin a fantasy of what may be one's economic situation. Seeing a clinician at church may also reveal religious or spiritual preferences. For clinicians who practice in rural states, these encounters may be frequent and almost expected as well as unavoidable.

Finally, there are self-disclosures that are a result of the reality of the Internet and the ease with which patients can discover personal information as a result of searching on the Web. Patients could even go further than looking at community service or resumes, which may be posted, and investigate any legal issues related to a clinician if they are willing to pay a fee. A clinician's marital history and past residences are on the Web for all to see, as well as other activities that may be entirely personal, such as committees served on and how long it took to run the local marathon. Clinicians ought to perform a search on themselves and know what is available to the public and learn to be selective about what to voluntarily post on the Internet.

The issue of when and what to disclose, in the category of deliberate self-disclosure, will be most fully explored in this discussion. I believe that for a novice clinician it presents real difficulty because talking about oneself would seem to provide a bridge to relationship building; the aim of patient-centered care. It is assumed that patients will be more comfortable if the clinician shares personal information. This line of thinking does not take into account the difference between a personal and professional relationship. One of the major differences between a personal and a professional relationship is the focus. In a personal relationship, ideally, the level of sharing or self-disclosure is balanced, otherwise one of the participants may feel slighted. If a friend or colleague shares a personal concern with you it may prompt you to reciprocate. However, in a professional relationship, the *patient* is the focus and so it is not a balanced relationship. When interacting with a patient the personal needs of the clinician ought not to be the focus. The very definition of nursing diagnosis, that of a patient's response to illness, is the appropriate focus of the interaction. When the conversation veers off to topics such as the latest movie or baseball score, it becomes social and not professional in nature. Particularly in an era of shortened clinical appointment times the focus needs to stay on the patient. While clinicians may be tempted to share their recent vacation or new restaurant find, it behooves patients for the clinician to stay focused on them.

Novice clinicians often fear that not sharing personal information will make them appear stiff, aloof, and cold, but forming a therapeutic relationship is about being empathetic, warm, genuine, and knowing how to listen. It is not about sharing your interest in sports or gardening. Staying on task, the task of the patient's concerns and responses to illness or health is the key. The statement that patients will be more comfortable if the clinician shares personal information is a classic case of projection. It is the clinician who may be more comfortable talking about the Red Sox rather than cancer, not the patient.

Therapeutic communication skills are complex, and conducting a therapeutic encounter takes energy and focus. It is tiring work. It is not surprising that if one overhears most communication in healthcare environments, whether it is the emergency room, the nursing home, the out-patient clinic, or the hospital, it is rife with personal self-disclosure on the part of staff. Many working with patients may simply not have training in how to communicate in a therapeutic and effective manner and others find it too difficult. In my graduate courses, when teaching nurses with decades of experience, it is not unusual for them to have to unlearn bad habits of relating and communicating. I am often shocked at what clinical encounters reveal in terms of inappropriate self-disclosure. Recently, my elderly mother had an initial visit from a visiting nurse for blood pressure checks 1 week after a hospitalization to stabilize her cardiac medications. These visits were scheduled twice weekly for a month. My mother had been quite frightened during the entire hospital stay, having suffered two prior heart attacks. When I asked her to tell me about the nursing home visit she proceeded to tell me a story of the nurse's teenage daughter who was pregnant. I asked my mother how she would know this and she relayed how the nurse, who she was meeting for the first time, expressed being upset and distracted by this event in her life. I could not help but think about all of the potential teaching moments that were lost in this interaction. In fact, the nurse never did get around to inquiring about my mother's reaction to the hospital stay or how she felt about being home. There was not enough time! It ended up being a visit to take and record a blood pressure, and to unload a personal concern on the part of the nurse. I cannot help but see this interaction as a missed opportunity to begin a therapeutic relationship, not burdened by personal issues.

Self-disclosure involves ethical issues because, if the sharing of personal information is not in the service of the patient, it is unethical. One concern is that the self-disclosure is more for the benefit of the clinician than the patient. In this instance the needs or desires of the clinician are met rather than those of the patient.

Keeping the patient in focus means putting personal concerns, worries, and stressors outside of the encounter. It also means refraining to launch into discussions about how one spends personal time just to be chatty or social. It also may mean deflecting personal questions that are asked during a clinical encounter. Personal questions always have an underlying agenda, and if a clinician simply answers a question, without seeking *why* it is being asked, a valuable piece of information may be lost. Take, for example, a simple question regarding marital status. If a patient asks if you are married, what is the patient really asking? It could be a number of issues in disguise. Is the patient concerned that if you are or are not married you will not understand a concern they have? It could be that they worry about trusting someone who is married or not married. It could mean that they would rather have you talk about yourself rather than the medical issue at hand. You will never know what is behind a question unless you inquire. So, "you are interested in my marital status?" will lead you to uncover what may be behind a seemingly innocuous inquiry.

One may ask if self-disclosure is ever appropriate. The litmus test is if, and only if, the self-disclosure is for a specific purpose related to assisting the patient. If the self-disclosure is based on patient welfare it falls into the category of beneficence or the intent to benefit the patient. If the information is related to the patient, that is patient focused and related to their concerns or treatment, or clinically driven. If the clinician can state the clinical purpose of the self-disclosure then it falls in the bounds of patient-centeredness and appropriate self-disclosure. These criteria will sort out much of the chatty banter that simply detracts from meaningful therapeutic communication in a clinical encounter.

Another classification of self-disclosures is provided by Servellen (2009) in Table 3-1.

Meta-disclosures are disclosures that refer to previous disclosures. These are process statements that refer to what is occurring in any communication rather than the content or what the topic of the communication contains. In a clinical interaction they may be useful when a provider is having trouble understanding what a patient is trying to communicate. Letting the patient know you do not understand their concerns or symptoms is a sort of self-disclosure about what they have shared and is entirely appropriate. It is patient focused and in the service of helping care for the patient.

Irresponsible disclosures are those made without considering the patient. They may be sharing that you or a family member have experienced a similar illness or symptom or life situation without having a specific goal that is patient-related in mind; therefore, they are inappropriate. Aggressive disclosures shared out of angry feelings on the part of the clinician may also fall into this category, as the intent is not to help the patient. While clinicians are human, and will

---

Table 3-1 Classification of Self-Disclosures

Type	Motivation
Meta-disclosures	Refer to previous disclosures
Irresponsible disclosures	Made without considering the patient
Manipulative disclosures	Made to manipulate patient into disclosing
Competitive disclosures	Made to appear superior to patient

experience frustration with patients, it is not an excuse for sharing these feelings with a patient.

Disclosures made in order to manipulate a patient into disclosing are also inappropriate. Threatening to discover a patient's illegal drug use if they do not disclose to you the truth may fall into this category. Really, any statement that pushes a patient to disclose more than they want to at any given moment can be considered to be manipulative and are to be avoided.

Finally, competitive disclosures do not have a place in a professional clinical encounter. The intent is to appear to be superior to the patient and, therefore, can serve no therapeutic value.

While the therapeutic value of self-disclosure has been investigated (Jourard, 1971), it is therapeutic only if it meets the important criteria of only disclosing what is the truth, with a clear therapeutic aim. This work, which identified the benefits of self-disclosure, including building trust, decreasing patient loneliness, lessening role distance, and establishing a sense of being, was written during a time when, culturally, power differentials in many areas of society were being rethought. One study (McDaniel et al., 2007) found that 85% of the time patients did not find self-disclosure of the provider to be helpful and, in fact, found them to be disruptive.

Guidelines have been suggested for identifying when self-disclosure might be useful to a provider (Auvil & Silver, 1984). These include:

1. Consideration of whether self-disclosure will enhance the patient's cooperation.
2. Consideration of whether self-disclosure will support or reinforce a patient's goals.
3. Consideration of whether self-disclosure will directly help a patient to deal with their problem.
4. Consideration of whether self-disclosure will help the patient to express feelings related to receiving emotional support.

These guidelines are quite subjective in nature and a provider must attempt to always be assured that the self-disclosure is in the service of the *patient* and their treatment. Self-disclosures that meet the needs of the provider must be avoided. Again, the hallmark of the professional therapeutic relationship is that the needs of the patient are paramount. Providers need to look elsewhere to meet their needs for socialization, relationship, and connection.

Self-disclosures are, at times, defended as being necessary to establish or maintain a therapeutic relationship. Novice clinicians may be concerned that by not answering personal questions or engaging in social chit chat that they may not be able to convey an interest in the patient. Rather than use self-disclosure, the health provider is advised to develop the skill of empathy in the clinical encounter.

In one interesting study, physician self-disclosure, defined as sharing personal experience that has medical or emotional relevance for a patient, was associated with higher patient satisfaction for surgical patient visits and lower satisfaction during primary care visits (Beach, Rubin, Frankel, Levinson, & Ford, 2004).

EMPATHY

There is no universal agreement on the definition of what empathy is. Some see it as more of a cognitive response to another's experience, and others see it as an emotional state of sharing feelings with another person. But this disagreement has not stopped the concept from being studied by scholars from a myriad of fields, including psychology, philosophy, and social and behavioral medicine. Empathy is usually compared to a similar but crucially different feeling, that of sympathy. The distinction between the two is important, in that while empathy is used to facilitate and enrich communication between clinician and patients, sympathy is both draining and not useful to either party. When experiencing sympathy for someone, the pain of the experience is *shared* and would therefore, in the professional sphere, render the provider incapable of being truly effective. Empathy, on the other hand, is a matter of imagining the experience of another, with a sense of engaged detachment. When imagining what the patient or family is experiencing, the clinician uses their experience to better understand the issues in order to provide intervention and treatment. This is also sometimes referred to as *participant observation*, in that the clinician is an active participant in the interaction while observing themselves and the patient at the same time. The value of empathy is not only communicating to the patient or family that one is a caring clinician, but it is also that the practice illuminates and guides intervention and treatment approaches.

Another way to understand empathy is to differentiate it from both sympathy and pity. Wilmer (1968) discusses all three emotions and notes that pity is often condescending and may involve the accompanying feelings of contempt on the part of the provider, while sympathy is shared suffering with little therapeutic value.

While it may be hard to define, clinicians intuitively know what empathy is and when they experience it in a clinical setting. They also may feel troubled when they cannot seem to muster it up when dealing with a particular patient or their family. The term has an interesting history, first described in 1873 by a German art historian, and was adopted by psychologists of the day to describe an aspect of human relationships. Freud incorporated the term in his model of psychodynamic treatment of neurosis and, ever since, social and behavioral theorists have studied the importance in provider–patient relationships (Hojat et al., 2002).

Fenichel (1945) believed that empathy was a process of first identifying with patients and then being aware of *both* their own feelings and those of the patient. It is the ability of trying to experience the situation that the patient is in, but also avoiding being stuck there. It requires the use of personal and professional boundaries to step outside of the situation, and be both connected and separate at the same time.

Educators have long debated whether empathy can be taught or if it is an inherent quality. The capacity for empathy seems to be a complex combination of one's temperament, early life experiences, motivations, and having a facilitating environment (Hojat et al., 2002). Empathy scales have been designed to test various groups, including the Hogan Empathy Scale, Mehrabian and Epstein's Emotional Empathy Scale, and Davis Interpersonal Reactivity Index. While none were developed exclusively for healthcare providers, they have served the purpose of health researchers who seek answers in this area of study. Empathy has been studied in relation to gender differences (Williams, 1989), personality (Miller & Eisenberg, 1988), and academic achievement (Colliver, Willis, Robbs, Cohen, & Swartz, 1998). It has also been studied in terms of the relationship between the existence of empathy and positive patient outcomes. It is clear that when an empathetic connection exists between a patient and their clinician, it results in an improved relationship and, therefore, has a positive effect on patient outcomes (Mercer & Reynolds, 2002). Stewart (1996) reviewed almost two dozen studies and found that there existed a positive correlation between physician–patient communications and health outcomes. One of the components of positive communications was empathetic engagement. Olson and Hanchett (1997) utilized the Orlando model of therapeutic relationships and found a significant relationship between nurses' empathy and positive patient outcomes. Orlando's focus in the nurse–patient interaction was on validation of what the patient was saying and feeling (Orlando, 1961). She developed communication strategies and techniques to help the clinician in fully understanding a patient's experience. These techniques have been a staple in undergraduate nursing when teaching about both communications and the nurse–patient relationship.

Empathy is usually differentiated from sympathy in that, when experiencing sympathy, the clinician may identify with the patient and feel sorry for them, in the form of pity. On the other hand, empathy is the ability to imagine what the patient is experiencing, in a cognitive way, and then express that understanding while maintaining an appropriate emotional barrier or boundary. This does not mean that clinicians do not experience feelings when hearing a sad story or experience as told by a patient. Yet, the ability to keep their feelings separate from those of the patient is key. If one has joined the patient emotionally then it is difficult to function in a useful or therapeutic fashion. A level of objectivity is required in order to assist the patient in dealing with what they are experiencing. It will not be useful to simply feel sorry for the patient or to convey one's similar experiences.

In one interesting study of empathy in physicians' responses to a patient's concern, "patients" were coached to raise the issue of chest pain in two different scenarios (McDaniel et al., 2007). In the first situation, chest pain was the primary symptom and, in the second, it represented a medically unexplained symptom. Patients asked whether the symptom of either chest pain or gastroesophageal reflux disease (GERD) might be "serious" and the physician response was recorded. Both a qualitative and quantitative study, researchers examined the responses in both types of clinical situations. This study, which involved 100 physicians, found that the most common responses were "redirecting" the patient toward "biomedical inquiry, action, medical explanation, and reassurance." Exploring the patient's feelings or psychosocial issues was uncommon when the symptom was medically unexplained, and even less so with patients presenting with GERD. The clinicians recommended diagnostic testing and medications or other treatments, usually later in the visit, and the expression of empathy occurred in only 15% of the visits, even after repeated prompting by the patient. The issue of providing reassurance was also studied by Dowrick, Ring, Humphris, and Salmon (2004) who found that when general practitioners used reassurance, the intervention was not only ineffective but also ran the risk of exacerbated the patient's presentation.

Patients often present with clues during a healthcare visit in the form of indirect or direct verbalizations about feelings or aspects of their life. These clues present an opportunity to demonstrate empathy and strengthen the relationship with the clinician. In a study of visits in primary care and surgery, patients initiated clues related to emotional issues connected to a medical condition or psychosocial issues 70% of the time and physicians responded to these cues about 30% of the time, regardless of setting (Levinson, Gorawara-Bhat, & Lamb, 2000). Opportunities to respond to patient clues were largely missed.

Platt and Kelley (1994) outlined the key steps to establishing empathy:

1. Identifying strong feelings such as anger, fear, grief, and disappointment in the clinical encounter
2. Pausing to imagine how the patient feels
3. Stating to the patient what the perception is of their feeling state in an effort to validate the feeling
4. Communicating an interest in working with the patient regarding the issues shared in the encounter

Each clinician must learn to find specific language which can deepen the conversation when strong emotions are expressed. Simple phrases will open up the dialogue and encourage the patient to share or elaborate an emotional reaction or issue, such as:

Tell me more.
How has that been for you?
What has that been like emotionally?

A clinician can use statements that are meant to clarify the patient's feelings and to communicate an interest in truly understanding the situation accurately, such as:

What I am hearing is . . .
Do I have this right?
Am I understanding you correctly?
Sounds like you are feeling . . .

One warning in these situations is to not lead the patient by introducing a feeling or response. If the clinician is careful to use the patient's words, the danger of influencing a patient who may wish to please a provider by simply agreeing with them will decrease.

While it is easy to extol the virtues of displaying empathy in the clinical encounter, there remain obstacles for clinicians in this area (Box 3-2).

COMPASSION FATIGUE

The concept of compassion fatigue is an evolving concept and is also referred to as *secondary traumatic stress, vicarious traumatization,* or *secondary victimization* (Figley, 2003). Although not currently an official listing in the *Diagnostic Statistical Manual* (*DSM IV*), it has caught the attention of clin-

---

Box 3-2   Obstacles for Clinicians

Not having sufficient time during a clinical visit
Finding the practice of expressing empathy to be emotionally draining
Fear of opening up difficult and sensitive topics
Insecurity in regard to having communication skills
Concern for spending one's emotional energy at work and not having any for one's family

icians and researchers alike. It has been studied in various groups of helpers including first responders, family members of traumatized veterans, and healthcare professionals. As the name would suggest, compassion fatigue relates to a disturbance in the usual compassion response from one person to another. Figley (2003) has outlined the process of compassion fatigue as beginning with exposure to suffering, followed by empathy, which can then revert to stress-related symptoms if the exposure is prolonged. Symptoms of compassion fatigue include feeling numb, withdrawn, irritable, and/or detached; experiencing anxiety or anxiety-related symptoms including intrusive memories of a patient or clinical incident; having difficulty sleeping; and overall negative, jaded or cynical feelings about life in general. A stress scale for secondary trauma has been developed by Bride (2004) that categorizes symptoms as avoidance, intrusion, or arousal. Cognitive changes include decreased concentration, forgetfulness, and apathy. Emotional changes include feelings of helplessness, anger, anxiety, and guilt. Behavioral changes include irritability and withdrawal and changes in sleep patterns and/or appetite. Spiritual changes include questioning the meaning of life and prior religious or spiritual beliefs. Work performance changes include decreased morale, avoiding certain tasks, poor productivity, and increased conflict with other staff (Jacobson, 2004).

A widely utilized self-test for compassion fatigue can be found in Stamm (1998). The survey offers professionals an objective way to assess their personal level of compassion fatigue as well as burnout.

In the literature, compassion fatigue is more closely aligned with trauma theory than the literature on burnout. In fact it differs from burnout in several important ways. Burnout symptoms include feelings of helplessness and overall difficulty with work or organizational issues. The onset is gradual and yet taking time off is often restorative (Wee & Myers, 2003).

Experiencing and displaying empathy can be both a rich, rewarding experience just as much as it can be emotionally taxing. The connection that can be made with patients and families is the very reason so many individuals enter health professions in the first place. To relegate practice to the mechanical aspects of providing health care robs professional life of the very essence of what it can be. In order to fully be present when working with patients, one must risk becoming emotionally affected. The key is to have sufficient boundaries which will form a protective barrier to the self. This does not mean being cold or detached, but rather, the ability to have appropriate emotional distance in order to keep the self intact and able to function in a professional capacity. Collaboration with other health team professionals has been cited as a preventative measure against compassion fatigue (Lindeke & Siekert, 2005). Joining a peer group for the purposes of debriefing as well as receiving support is a proven antidote to compassion fatigue. Acknowledging unexpressed grief has also been cited as an important process in terms of preventing compassion fatigue (Meadors & Lamson, 2008). An interesting qualitative study found that nurses who were able to utilize moments of connection with patients were able to avoid experiencing compassion fatigue (Perry, 2008). Other research points to the clinician developing specific coping mechanisms as well as building and maintaining a solid support system (Matum, Heiman, & Garwick, 2004).

In addition to the use of boundaries, the clinician must have a rewarding personal life away from the workplace that is both rewarding and nurturing. At the end of a difficult day, or week, it is critical that one can retreat to a myriad of activities that nurture the soul. Whether it is yoga, gardening, reading, listening to music, watercolors, jewelry making, kickboxing, or jogging, the issue is one of finding activities that nurture the self. In this way clinicians will be recharged and able to deal with the emotional demands of parenting, being in intimate relationships, or caring for elderly parents. If one is able to recharge one's emotional batteries, then returning to the clinical area fully present is possible. Standing with patients and families, positioned as a caring human being, is possible. If this can be achieved then the need to retreat emotionally lessens and clinical practice remains genuine and rich because the clinician is able to connect to patients and families. Having a full and rich personal life is not only necessary to prevent compassion fatigue, it is also necessary if one is to sustain one's practice with the powerful tool of empathy.

COMMUNICATION EXERCISES

1. Boundary Violation

Pair off as patient and provider: 30 minutes.

Provider:

Conduct an initial assessment of a patient.

Patient:

Challenge your provider by pushing boundaries in some manner. Ask highly personal questions, be seductive, or both.

Continue this behavior throughout the clinical encounter.

Discussion:

Assess together the effectiveness of the responses of the provider.

If less than effective, what suggestions do you have for alternative responses in this type of clinical situation?

Share with each other any experiences that you have had with patients pushing your boundaries.

Identify how you dealt with these situations and what thoughts you have about managing them in the future.

_____

_____

_____

_____

_____

_____

_____

_____

2. Self-Disclosure

Triad of provider, patient, and observer/recorder: 45 minutes.

Provider:

Respond to the patient utilizing therapeutic communication techniques of redirection, refocusing, and commenting on process.

Patient:

You are shopping for a primary care provider. After your examination (annual physical) you pepper the provider with personal questions. Be overly personal, intrusive, and deliberately cross boundaries.

Observer:

Evaluate how the provider fared. Did they seem defensive? Did they effectively use refocusing and redirection?

Switch all three roles.

Discussion:

What were the challenges of a patient who asks personal questions?

What worked and what seemed to backfire?

How did it feel as a patient for the clinician to use the techniques?

What body language did the observer notice?

What suggestions do you have for managing this situation in the future?

_____

_____

_____

_____

_____

_____

_____

_____

3. Reassurance

Pair off as patient and provider: 30 minutes.

Provider:

You know that this 59-year-old patient was recently widowed, and presents to the clinic for her annual physical. When she describes her feelings of sadness, be overly reassuring to her. Do not let her fully describe her feelings, rather, be reassuring.

Patient:

You are a 59-year-old woman who has experienced the death of her husband after 35 years of marriage. You have been very sad and lost interest in your usual hobbies. Your children are impatient with you and, after 6 months, you have stopped sharing your feelings with them. You are worried about telling your primary care provider how you really feel during your routine annual physical exam.

Discussion:

The patient should share with the provider what it was like to receive reassurances.

Switch roles and repeat.

_____

_____

_____

_____

_____

_____

_____

4. Giving Advice versus Information

Pair off as patient and provider: 30 minutes.

Provider:

In the first half of the interview, respond to the patient with advice about her situation. Use statements such as "If it were me . . ." or "I think you should . . . ."

In the second half of the interview, do not give advice but, rather, give information in regard to this issue.

Patient:

You are a 29-year-old woman who has become increasingly concerned about her biological clock. You want to discuss this with your primary care provider.

Discussion:

As the provider, how comfortable were both responses in this clinical encounter?

As the patient, share with your provider what both parts of the interview felt like.

Switch roles and repeat.

_____

_____

_____

_____

_____

_____

_____

_____

5. Various Types of Disclosure

Pair off as patient and provider: 1 hour.

Provider:

In the course of an intake interview, demonstrate examples of the various types of disclosure (deliberate, accidental, unavoidable, or as a result of client action) in four separate interactions.

Patient:

Respond to each of the disclosures as you might imagine a patient might during a clinical encounter.

Discussion:

Compare and contrast as provider and patient the reactions to the different disclosures.

Were any helpful?

Did any make you uncomfortable? If so, why?

Discuss the insight you might have gained from this exercise.

Switch roles and repeat.

_____
_____
_____
_____
_____
_____
_____
_____

6. Empathy

Pair off as patient and provider: 30 minutes.

Provider:

As you conduct the interview, pay attention to your inner responses to this patient.

Patient:

Develop a presenting problem or life story that might make it difficult for a provider to experience empathy.

Discussion:

Provider:

What about this patient made feeling empathy difficult?

How did you display this to the patient, if at all?

How did you manage your feelings during the encounter?

What were you tempted to do after the interview ended?

How does this experience inform you about yourself?

Patient:

Were you aware of any difference in response from the provider?

Discuss your experience of this provider.

Provide feedback to your provider for future encounters.

Switch roles and repeat.

_____

_____

_____

_____

_____

_____

_____

_____

7. Empathy Challenges

Pair off as patient and provider: 30 minutes.

Provider:

Conduct a typical consultation with a patient you are seeing for the first time.

Patient:

Present to the clinic with vague symptoms and be a poor historian.

Discussion:

Provider:

Examine the display of empathy with this patient.

How did you attempt to display this to your patient? Give examples.

Were there any challenges?

Do you think you were successful? If so, why? If not, explain.

Give a summary and analysis of this interaction with empathy as the focal point.

Patient:

Provide feedback to the provider in terms of your experience of feeling understood.

What displays of empathy did you receive? Be specific.

How did your provider fare in terms of coming across as empathetic?

What suggestions might you have for your provider?

Switch roles and repeat.

_____

_____

_____

_____

_____

_____

_____

_____

8. Clues in the Clinical Encounter

Pair off as patient and provider: 30 minutes.

Provider:

Respond to your patient's presenting symptoms. Utilize therapeutic communication skills.

Patient:

Develop a scenario in which you present with several symptoms and also with clues about an emotional issue or psychosocial concern in your life.

Discussion:

Did the provider pick up on the underlying issue?

If so, how effective was their response (patient's perspective)?

What was the internal experience of the provider?

Compare the two experiences and discuss the implications for expressing empathy and deepening the therapeutic relationship.

Discuss how you might incorporate sensitivity to patient clues in your practice at present and in the future.

Switch roles and repeat.

JOURNALING EXERCISES

1. Who are You?

Develop a statement regarding your personal philosophy of care that you will wish to communicate to new patients who may be looking for a provider.

What do you say about what is important to you?

Do you make it clear what patients can expect of you?

Do you articulate what you expect of patients?

After writing this statement, practice it out loud.

Practice this statement with peers and receive feedback when they play the role of a perspective patient.

Amend the statement according to peer feedback.

_____

_____

_____

_____

_____

_____

_____

_____

2. Your Personal and Professional Self

How do you describe the differences between your personal and professional self?

Is there a great distance between the two?

What qualities of your personal self do you want to incorporate into a professional persona?

What qualities do you want to keep separate?

What qualities of yourself tend to overlap in regard to a personal and professional identity?

Do you consider yourself on the warm or chilly side of the emotional spectrum?

What are the advantages and disadvantages of this, both personally and professionally?

Do you consider yourself to be a logical and cognitively oriented person?

What are the advantages and disadvantages of this, both personally and professionally?

What are your goals for personal and professional self-improvement?

Which goals are separate and which are the same?

Discuss this with a peer.

_____

_____

_____

_____

_____

_____

_____

_____

3. Acceptance

Which illnesses or presenting complaints might generate emotions that make acceptance of the patient difficult?

Write about a recent patient or family who challenged your ability to be nonjudgmental and accepting.

Describe the clinical encounter with a focus on your acceptance.

Was the patient's attitude difficult to accept?

What are your associations to this behavior?

Did you adequately explore this behavior with the patient? If not, why not?

Explore an alternative response on your part to the patient or family.

_____

_____

_____

_____

_____

_____

_____

_____

4. Responsiveness

Recall a clinical encounter in which you were responsive to a subtle cue from a patient or family.

What was the indirect or incomplete message you responded to?

Was the cue a gesture, tone of voice, or hesitation on the part of the patient?

How exactly did you convey your responsiveness to the patient?

_____

_____

_____

_____

_____

_____

_____

_____

5. Clinician Anxiety

What types of patients or clinical situations cause you to experience anxiety?

What is your understanding of this?

Recall a recent clinical encounter that made you anxious.

What were the specifics of the encounter?

How did your anxiety affect the clinical encounter?

What might you do differently in future with this type of patient?

_____

_____

_____

_____

_____

_____

_____

_____

6. Preoccupation

Write about a time when your personal life interfered with your ability to listen to a patient's story.

How do you usually manage personal stress?

What resources are available for you to process personal issues?

In general do you find separating your personal issues and professional life to be challenging?

How would you like to manage these issues in your practice?

_____

_____

_____

_____

_____

_____

_____

_____

7. Mirroring Encounters

Describe a recent clinical encounter with a patient or family that closely mirrored a situation occurring in your own life.

How did this parallel situation affect your ability to communicate effectively?

What are the changes you might make in another clinical encounter that mirrors your personal life?

_____

_____

_____

_____

_____

_____

_____

_____

8. Giving Advice

Do an experiment today during any encounter with a friend. Practice listening without giving any advice.

How difficult was this for you?

What other skills did you have to use during the encounter?

Write about any other thoughts regarding advice-giving.

Do you find not giving advice too easy or challenging in the clinical setting?

Does not giving advice create anxiety for you?

How do you define advice giving and providing information to patients?

_____

_____

_____

_____

_____

_____

_____

_____

9. Self-Disclosure

Write about an experience of bumping into a current or former patient in a social setting.

How did you feel about seeing the patient?

If with others, how did you manage questions about who this was?

How did you handle the interaction?

Was it awkward at all?

Did the conversation get personal?

How might you handle this experience in future?

If you have not had such an experience, write about how you wish to handle this type of experience.

Identify any other encounters of accidental self-disclosure you might have had.

_____

_____

_____

_____

_____

_____

_____

_____

_____

10. Empathy

Define the differences between empathy and sympathy in clinical interventions with patients and families.

Describe a recent clinical encounter where you effectively communicated in an empathetic manner.

What was the particular clinical situation and setting?

Now describe a clinical encounter where you could not muster up an empathetic response to a patient or family.

What were the particulars of this encounter?

Describe what your reaction was to the patient or family.

What interfered with your ability to be empathetic?

What can be learned from this clinical encounter that can inform your practice in future?

What additional feelings are generated in you as a clinician when you do not find an empathetic connection to a patient?

Share with a peer.

_____

_____

_____

_____

_____

_____

_____

11. Boundaries

Imagine a situation of a patient you are caring for asks you out for a date. You are both single and available—is there an issue?

What are the ethical implications of crossing this line?

What are the legal implications for doing so?

How tempting would this situation be for you if the patient was very attractive to you and you had a lot in common?

Is there ever a statute of limitations on this once you are not treating the patient?

Discuss the issue of power differentials and relationships and how that concept might apply to the patient–provider relationship.

Do you know of any friend who is a clinician and experienced this dilemma? How did they handle the situation?

Do you have any particular concerns about your managing this situation?

What resources do you have for discussing your thoughts about this?

_____

_____

_____

_____

_____

_____

_____

12. Competitive Self-Disclosure

Have you ever felt a sense of competition with a patient?

Describe the patient and your relationship with them.

In what area did the issue of being competitive arise?

How was the issue displayed in a clinical encounter?

When were you aware of the issue of competition with this patient?

What ideas do you have of handling this encounter differently?

What effect do you think your being competitive had for the relationship with the patient?

Do you consider yourself to be a competitive person in general?

What have been your positive experiences with competition in your life?

How do you think the issue of competitiveness will play out in your clinical practice in the future?

What resources do you have for discussing this issue if it should arise in your clinical work?

_____

_____

_____

_____

_____

_____

_____

_____

13. Compassion Fatigue

After taking the self-test, discuss whether you are at risk for developing compassion fatigue.

What symptoms of compassion fatigue have you ever experienced?

List your current methods of dealing with work stress.

How would you assess the effectiveness of your current methods?

What are you willing to consider in terms of building coping skills?

Describe an encounter with a colleague who you believe is experiencing compassion fatigue.

Explore your concerns for yourself in this area.

What is your knowledge of peer groups? Assess your ability to start and participate in such a group.

_____

_____

_____

_____

_____

_____

_____

_____

14. Personal–Professional Boundaries

How would you define your personal and professional boundaries?

Where in your past did you learn about boundaries?

What lessons did you learn from your family-of-origin in regard to boundaries?

Describe any challenges you have in this area in terms of your personal or professional life.

How do you manage to address these challenges?

Describe how these efforts affect your work with patients in a clinical setting.

REFERENCES

Auvil, C. A, & Silver, B. W. (1984). Therapist self-disclosure. *Perspectives of Psychiatric Care*, *22*(2), 57–61.

Beach, M. C., Rubin, H., Frankel, R., Levinson, W., & Ford, D. E. (2004). Is physician self-disclosure related to patient evaluation of office visits? *Journal of General Medicine*, *9*(9), 6.

Bride, B. (2004). Development and validation of the secondary traumatic stress scale. *Research on Social Work Practice*, *14*(1), 27–35.

Colliver, J. A., Willis, M. S., Robbs, R. S., Cohen, D. S., & Swartz, M. H. (1998). Assessment of empathy in a standardized-patient examination. *Teaching and Learning in Medicine*, *10*, 3.

Dowrick, C., Ring, A., Humphris, G., & Salmon, P. (2004). Normalisation of unexplained symptoms by general practitioners: a functional typology. *British Journal of General Practice*, *54*(500), 165–170.

Fenichel, O. (1945). *The psychoanalytic theory of neurosis*. New York: W. W. Norton.

Figley, C. (2003). *Compassion fatigue*. Tallahassee, FL: Green Cross Foundation.

Hojat, M., Gonella, J. S., Nasca, T. J., Mangione, S., Vergare, M., & Magee, M. (2002). Physician empathy: definition, components, measurement, and relationship to gender and speciality. *American Journal of Psychiatry*, *159*, 1563–1569.

Jacobson, J. M. (2004). Preventing compassion fatigue and promoting compassion satisfaction. Available at http://www.easpassn/public/articles/compassionfatigue.pdf. Accessed August 7, 2009.

Jourard, D. (1971). *The transparent self.* New York: Van Nostrand Reinhold.

Levinson, W., Gorawara-Bhat, R., & Lamb, J. (2000). A study of patient clues and physician responses in primary care and surgical settings. *Journal of the American Medical Association, 284,* 1021–1027.

Lindeke, L., & Sieckert, A. M. (2005). Nurse-physician workplace collaboration. *Online Journal of Issues in Nursing, 10*(1), 1–6.

Matum, J. C., Heiman, M. B., & Garwick, A.W. (2004). Compassion fatigue and burnout in nurses who work with children with chronic conditions and their families. *Journal of Pediatric Health Care, 18*(4), 171–179.

Makoul, G., & Strauss, A. (2003). Building therapeutic relationships during patient visits. *Journal of General Internal Medicine, 18*(Suppl.1), 275.

Meadors, P., & Lamson, A. (2008). Compassion fatigue and secondary traumatization: Provider self care on intensive care units for children. *Journal of Pediatric Health Care, 22,* 24–34.

McDaniel, S. H., Beckman, H. B., Morse, D., Silberman, J., Seaburn, D. B., & Epstein, R. (2007). Physician self-disclosure in primary care visits. *Archives of Internal Medicine, 167*(12), 6.

Mercer, S. W., & Reynolds, W. (2002). Empathy and quality of care. *British Journal of General Practice, 52,* 4.

Miller, P., & Eisenberg, N. (1988).The relation between empathy and aggressive and externalizing/antisocial behavior. *Psychological Bulletin, 103,* 20.

Olson, J., & Hanchett, E. (1997). Nurse-expressed empathy, patient outcomes, and development of a middle-range theory. *Image, 29,* 6.

Orlando, I. (1961).*The dynamic nurse-patient relationship.* New York: Putnam.

Perry, B. (2008). Why exemplary oncology nurses seem to avoid compassion fatigue. *Canadian Oncolology Nursing Journal, 18,* 87–99.

Platt, F., & Kelley, V. (1994). Empathic communication: a teachable and learnable skill. *Journal of General Internal Medicine, 9*(4), 5.

Stewart, M. A. (1996). Effective physician-patient communication and health outcomes. *Canadian Medical Association Journal, 152,* 10.

Servellen, G. (2009). *Communication skills for the health care professional* (2nd ed.) Sudbury, MA: Jones and Bartlett.

Stamm, B. H. (1998). *Measures of traumatic stress and secondary traumatic stress.* Retrieved May 13, 2009 from http://www.isu.edu/;bhstamm/tests.htm.

The Treehouse. (2006). Professional boundaries in health-care relationships. Retrieved May 13, 2009 from http://www.survivors-treehouse.net

Wee, D., & Myers, D. (2003). Compassion satisfaction, compassion fatigue, and critical incident stress management. *International Journal of Emergency Mental Health, 5*(1), 33–37.

Williams, C. A. (1989). Empathy and burnout in male and female helping professionals. *Research in Nursing & Health,* 12, 9.

Wilmer, H. A. (1968). The doctor-patient relationship and issues of pity, sympathy and empathy. *British Journal of Medical Psychology, 41*(3), 243–248.

Zur, O. (2008). The Google factor: Therapists' self-disclosure in the age of the Internet: Discover what your clients can find out about you with a click of the mouse. *The Independent Practitioner, 28*(2), 82–85.

SUGGESTED READINGS

Hardee, J. T. (2003 Fall). An overview of empathy. *The Permanente Journal, 7*(7). Retreived May 13, 2009 from http://xnet.kp.org/permanentejournal/fall03/cpc.html

Maslach, C. (1982). *Burnout: The cost of caring.* Upper Saddle River, NJ: Prentice-Hall.

Platt, F. W. (1992). Empathy: can it be taught? *Annals of Internal Medicine, 117*(8), 1.

Suchman, A. L., Markakis, K., Beckman, H. B., & Frankel, R. (1997). A model of empathic communication in the medical interview. *JAMA, 277*(8), 5.

CHAPTER 4

The Art of Listening

Valerie A. Hart

It is more important to know what sort of person has a disease than to know what sort of disease a person has.

—Hippocrates

If migraine patients have a common and legitimate second complaint besides their migraines, it is that they have not been listened to by physicians. Looked at, investigated, drugged, charged, but not listened to.

—Dr. Oliver Sacks, British neurologist

ACTIVE LISTENING

There is concern expressed among those who educate clinicians about how to prepare their students to meet the rigorous demands of today's healthcare environment. Some argue that, in an attempt to prepare students to be *professional*, educators stress rules and procedures rather than the very *personal* side of providing care (Coulehan, 2005). It indeed can be argued that the virtues of caring and relating to patients take a backseat to the demands of staying on a tight schedule or filling out paperwork. The challenge of listening, really listening, to patients requires specific skills, intense focus, emotional energy, and solid commitment to the task. Listening in an active and therapeutic manner is the foundational skill for any clinician. It differs dramatically from the sort of listening many do in social situations and settings. This is not to say that the skill of active listening is not of value in one's personal life. In fact, learning these skills will enrich both personal and professional relationships.

Perhaps the reason adults only retain 25% of what they hear is due to the notion that listening is a passive activity. Our ability to speak lags far behind our ability to think, in terms of speed, and perhaps it explains the common trap of jumping ahead of what another is saying. Other explanations include the emotional factors that play a part in conversations, and sometimes the need for the listener to mount a sound defense. If the listener is attending to their response, they can not fully listen because their mind is literally elsewhere. Words are inadequate communication tools, due to differing interpretations of words. It is so easy to misinterpret what another is saying, even when paying attention and not drifting off in our own head.

Conversation is an active activity in which joint understanding of what the other person means is important. When one person is not able to clearly understand the other's words, then miscommunication, misunderstanding, and perhaps negative consequences can occur. For example, in one study, listening to recorded instructions resulted in over eight times as many errors as opposed to in-person instructions (Clark & Krych, 2004). This should be a concern for practitioners whose practice is telephone-based consultation. This format clearly exposes clinicians to a liability not previously experienced in practice. Marvel, Epstein, Flowers, and Beckman (1999) found that patients are often redirected after stating their original concerns and, once redirected, the descriptions are rarely completed. Subsequently, patients bring up additional concerns late in the visit, when there may be inadequate time to fully assess the issue. Therefore, the wisdom of interrupting patients during the beginning of the clinical visit may, in fact, backfire. Greer and Halgin (2006) discovered that physicians and patients agreed on the etiology of symptoms only 59% of the time, and patients who disagreed were seen as less cooperative.

As clinicians we listen in order to accurately assess, which leads to accurate treatment. The data from malpractice lawsuits inform us that behaviors that lead to judgments against registered nurses include failure to educate, to intervene, to recognize symptoms, and overall inadequate communication among staff. Nurse practitioners' malpractice fees are increasing and insurers are finding the business of insuring advanced practice nurses to be less profitable due to increasing lawsuits. Attending to communication skills has never been more important.

Awareness of nonverbal communication plays a part in active listening. Facial expressions, body position, and posture all communicate in a powerful way. Preparing for a clinical encounter means being conscious about where and how you sit or stand in the room. It means paying attention to eye contact with the patient or family members. It also means purposely using hand gestures and facial movements. Think of your last visit to a primary care provider. Recall the greeting you received from both the assistant and the provider. Was it personal or impersonal? Did the provider have their eyes buried in your chart or did they make eye contact with you? Did they remain standing or sitting and what was the height of the provider in relation to you? What facial expressions were exhibited by the provider during the interaction? How did any of these behaviors affect the quality of the interaction?

In a clinical encounter a provider must rely on the skills of being an *active* listener. In the encounter there are no clinical guidelines or protocols for reference. Each patient will present unique challenges that may differ a great deal from patients that are described in a textbook. The initial contact with a patient will set the tone for the entire provider–patient relationship, one that may extend over many years. In an initial contact, which may have a diagnostic focus, the patient and/or their family will also be assessing our communication skills and making decisions regarding their ability to form a relationship. While novice clinicians will undoubtedly feel self-conscious about their ability to relate to and effectively communicate with patients, there are guidelines for increasing the potential for a therapeutic encounter. It is natural to wonder about our ability to listen with all our senses, or have an ability to understand the patient. It is healthy to be aware of any tendency to be judgmental or critical when hearing someone's health narrative. It is understandable to have a concern about our ability to be empathetic and helpful to the patient or family. The techniques taught in a textbook are only a guide, as the outcome of every clinical situation will depend on many variables. A foundational variable is the ability to listen in an active manner.

Active listening is a skill that can be taught. It is clear that when clinicians realize the benefit of perfecting this skill, they can improve performance in this area (Butterworth, 2004). Even seasoned clinicians can work on improving this skill as a result of reflection and practice, and in clinical supervision. While it is clear that active listening is a vital skill in nonclinical areas in an organization, its use in the clinical setting will be our focus.

In a study of primary care physicians' responses to patients when they present with vague symptoms, researchers found that the physicians usually ignored the ambiguity and became more directive (Seaburn, McDaniel, Beckman, Silberman, & Epstein, 2005). Fewer physician responses consisted of exploring the patient's concerns and exploring the ambiguity, therefore engaging the patient and relating to their perspective of their issues.

THE STEPS OF ACTIVE LISTENING

Clearing Your Mind

The first step in this process is one of mental preparation (Table 4-1). It requires that you clear your mind. This means not thinking of the patient you have just seen, or the one you have scheduled later in the day, as well as thoughts of your personal life. Anyone who has even practiced meditation can relate to

Table 4-1   The Steps of Active Listening

Clear your mind	Similar to meditation; let distracting thoughts drift away; focus on current patient only; use breathing control to focus
Get on the same page	Use the following techniques to ensure you understand your patient: Restate patient's statements Paraphrase patient's words in your own Clarify by asking questions
Reflect on the issue	Use your observational skills, along with the patient's statements, to dig deeper and show you understand the patient's perspective
Validate and summarize	Provide feedback and information; individualized care; can include intervention and treatment planning

how difficult it is to empty one's mind. Thoughts keep developing and can lead us into interesting and distracting places if not curbed. When one is in the professional role, this is particularly important. Attempt to clear your mind, as one would start with a fresh canvas when beginning a new painting. Although distracting thoughts may arise, do not let them latch on in your mind but, rather, let them drift away. Practice a brief meditative exercise just before meeting with a patient or family that clears the mind. Breathwork is another practice that can serve to clear the mind and prepare for an upcoming encounter. It is also a useful tool when having to go from one clinical encounter to another in a short amount of time. It does not require special equipment or a special setting. First, close your eyes, and take in a deep breath. Count to four, then exhale to the count of four, hold to the count of four, and repeat. This simple yet effective technique is a way of rebooting your breathing pattern, slowing the breath, and is particularly helpful when one is feeling anxious. It has an overall calming effect on the mind and body, and is the perfect preparation for any new situation.

Getting on the Same Page

Now that you are ready to begin to listen, the techniques of *paraphrasing, restating, clarification, reflection,* and *validation* are utilized. Remember that one of the most important goals of any patient interaction, but particularly true if it is a new relationship, is to have the patient feel that they are understood. Because of the difficulty of language and words, it requires communication techniques that continually try to assure that what the patient is saying and what you understand is the same thing. The only way to know this for sure is to ask for clarity, to repeat in your own words what the patient is saying, and to summarize both the issue and the feelings associated with the issue. At times you will be repeating what the patient has said, and at other times making a statement and asking the patient if you are correct in making a connection. The process repeats until you hear the magic words from the patient: "exactly."

One of the most powerful, and yet seemingly simple, methods in this process is to use the patient's own words. The technique of repeating the patient's last two words, with a questioning tone or using a fill-in-the-blank format, can be very effective. The important thing is to stay with the patient's words and concerns and not skip to another topic, which can feel dismissive to the patient. For example, the patient says, "I have been so worried about my son." Following with "your son?" will encourage the patient to expand on the topic. Even saying, "Why are you worried?" while perhaps an attempt to be supportive and therapeutic, can be perceived as putting the patient on the spot. The patient may not be clear about why they are worried, or may read some judgment (real or not) in the question. It might take a dialogue for the patient to get at the heart of the worry, so the aim is to open up the dialogue.

Restatement of the patient's concern or paraphrasing in your own words is the beginning step to making sure you and the patient are on the same page. Overuse of this might become annoying to the patient, as if you are doing nothing but parroting their words, so varying techniques is suggested. However, the use of these techniques communicates to a patient or family that you are interested in getting it right, interested in their concerns, and interested in them. It says you are paying attention to the individual, and that is the essence of patient-centered care. The patient has the opportunity to hear what message the clinician is receiving. It empowers patients to correct us and builds the relationship as a result of the interactive nature of the process. For the clinician, the techniques of paraphrasing and restating also keep us on track, and make us less prone to get sidetracked from the business going on in our mind. The patient always needs to be the focus of the communication and this tool helps to serve that purpose.

Paraphrasing is simply reflecting back to the patient *in your words* what you understand them to be saying. It is similar to restatement, but with more of the clinician's wording. In paraphrasing one might use the preface of "It sounds like," "What I am hearing is," or "Let me see if I have it right." A combination of restatement and paraphrasing is typical in an exchange, as they both accomplish the same thing.

Clarification is a technique utilized if an aspect of what the patient has said is contradictory or confusing. You may need to ask about how long the patient has been experiencing a symptom or for details about any aspect of what the patient has said. Either closed-ended or open-ended questions can be utilized throughout a therapeutic dialogue, with an emphasis on the latter—always allow the patient to tell you their story rather than answer "yes" or "no," which closes off the dialogue.

Once things are clear, they can be summarized for the patient and offered in order to get validation that the clinician really understands the issues. Continue to use clarification until you are confident you understand exactly what the patient is communicating. Refining your clarifying statements until the patient says "exactly" is the goal. This may seem tedious, but is actually a time-saver considering that inquiring about an incorrect or irrelevant issue is a waste of time. Staying on track with the patient and communicating your expertise as well as interest in them can be accomplished by repeated uses of restatement, paraphrasing, and clarification.

Reflecting on the Issue

Now the clinician can offer a statement regarding how the patient is feeling about the symptom or issue. This is also done in the service of attempting to understand, from the patient's perspective. This step of the process of active listening is more intuitive than the previous steps. It also depends more on a clinician's experience. Reflecting on the issue is an opportunity to read between the words of what the patient is saying or not saying. Use of body language, observational skills, your knowledge of the patient, and your personality all play a critical role in this skill. More important than "getting it right" is the effort made by the provider to dig deeper than the superficial presentation of complaints with which the patient presents. Offering a possible feeling or attitude without a need to be right is a matter of simply offering a possible reality. The clinician can state it with a questioning tone and the patient is free to agree or not, which will further lead to other areas of discussion.

As a couples' psychotherapist, miscommunication is almost always present when a couple is in distress. For years I have utilized a simple exercise of one person stating a concern while the other listens and is not allowed to speak. That is often challenging because people are so accustomed to defending themselves that not being allowed to do so is foreign. The next step is for the party with the concern to state it in one sentence. It requires that the individual boils down their complaint and that they focus on what is really the heart of the matter. The respondent is then allowed to repeat back what their partner has said.

As simple as it seems, I have frequently spent extended periods of time with helping a couple accomplish this step. The misunderstanding of what is being said is often profound, and listening without making assumptions is not a skill we often practice in our relationships. This is especially true if the relationship is full of conflict or there are strong emotions involved.

Learning to listen instead of talking is much harder than it seems. In the professional arena it takes on a whole new meaning as one develops an understanding of how communication and listening differ in one's personal and professional lives. The flow of words and concepts is different, as well as the pace of the conversation. It requires developing a comfort level in the area of silences in conversation.

In a social conversation the sudden appearance of silence can feel quite awkward. Tension builds as both parties search for the next words. There is a sense that something is off, and both may scramble to fill the void. However in a therapeutic encounter, use of silence is a powerful technique. It is to be welcomed, rather than avoided. Much can be learned if only one has the discipline and patience to *not* fill the space with words. The important part is not to disconnect from the patient, by shifting position or breaking eye contact. Staying in connection and remaining silent will communicate that you expect the patient to keep talking and it will surprise you where the patient may take the conversation. There can be a deepening of the current topic, or the introduction of an entirely new topic that may be related by association. This is the classic strategy of letting patient's *free associate* in therapy. Too often a practitioner's own anxiety will prevent them from allowing the space of the silence to expand. Rich opportunities are lost if this occurs.

When practicing the skill of the therapeutic use of silence, attend to your breath and gently pinch the inside of your cheek as a reminder to not talk. The payoff from developing this skill will be reinforcing for the clinician and soon this technique will become easier and easier in a clinical encounter.

The step of reflecting on feelings without a two-way flow of information marks a departure from the manner in which personal communication occurs. Instead of sharing your feelings, as one does with a friend or relative, the clinician stays with the patient's concerns.

Validating and Summarizing

In this part of the interaction, the clinician provides both feedback to the patient about how they understand the patient's concerns, in a summation, and shares their reaction to the situation. It may have an educational component, as the clinician informs or instructs the patient about misconceptions or places the clinical situation in a larger context. For example, if the patient is highly worried about a relatively common or minor issue, the clinician can provide information that may help the patient to see the issue with a different perspective. If the patient or family has read information derived from an Internet search, the clinician may need to make corrections or expand on what the patient has researched. Some patients will welcome direction in finding credible Web sites and will eagerly ask for more information. Other patients may need simple and clear instructions and information and will not be interested in other health-related resources.

This step requires individualizing care and having a sense of what might be most useful to the patient at this time. Overloading a patient or family with too much information is always a danger, as is the danger of not providing enough knowledge of an illness or condition. From the first minutes of the clinical encounter, the provider ought to be sizing up the patient and family in regard to their health literacy. What is the appropriate level of information this patient might need? What is the motivational level of this patient or family at the present time? How much does this patient seem to know at this point in regard to this condition? Where do they usually receive their health information? How does this patient regard health in their overall priority list?

After determining these factors, the provider can proceed in terms of intervention and treatment planning. Active listening is the method of making sure you genuinely understand the patient's concerns and symptoms. Providing validation and then summary of the situation can either lead to the patient feeling a sense of reassurance or to more concern, based on the findings.

Proceeding with different populations will be taken up in various sections of the text. Much has been written about in terms of gender differences and communication (Coates, 1986; Glass, 1992; Tannen, 1990). Regardless of the specific characteristics of the individual patient, active listening is required. Additional skills will be required if the patient is a child, adolescent, or elder. However, the foundation for all communication is the ability to truly listen and hold back the temptation to talk too much instead of listen to patients.

SPECIFIC ISSUES IN ADVANCED PRACTICE AND PRIMARY CARE INTERRUPTIONS

Clinicians in primary care settings often feel a time crunch of seeing patients in a very tight schedule. Time management in ambulatory patient visits is increasingly critical. An interesting study, perhaps a counterintuitive one, revealed that allowing a patient to complete their monologue without interruption only slightly lengthens the monologue, but *shortens* the overall consultation time

(Rabinowitz, Tamir, & Reis, 2004). There is plenty of evidence that specific interventions can affect patient communication in a positive manner (Rao, Inui, & Frankel, 2007). Studies have examined the issue of interruptions that occur between patients and providers (Rhoades, Finch, & Johnson, 2001; Langewitz et al., 2002), revealing that patients are interrupted rapidly (ranging from 12–22 seconds) when trying to convey the reason for a patient care visit. In addition, patients speak less than clinicians in a typical patient visit, leading one to draw the conclusion that learning to listen to patients is a skill that still needs to be taught and practiced. Beyond verbal interruptions on the part of clinicians, telephone calls during a visit present another problem and only 40% of patients in their study felt that the physician gave them "undivided" attention during the visit (Urkin et al., 2002.)

Time Constraints

In one literature review, three strategies were found to be effective in addressing concerns about time constraint in primary care (Mauksch et al., 2008). These include rapport building, agenda setting, and the acknowledgement of patient clues regarding emotional issues. Haidet and Paterniti (2003) recommend a "narrative" approach with an emphasis on "information sharing" during the clinical interview. A systematic review of encounters in primary care found that certain behaviors positively associated with health outcomes included empathy, reassurance and support, explanations, positive reinforcement, humor, psychosocial talk, health education, friendliness, courtesy, orienting the patient during examination, and summarization and clarification (Beck, Daughtridge, & Sloane, 2002). Nonverbal behaviors positively associated with outcomes included head nodding, forward lean, direct body orientation, uncrossed legs and arms, arm symmetry, and less mutual gaze.

Relationships Over Time

Providing health care in a primary care setting, as opposed to an inpatient hospital setting, presents both challenges and opportunities in the area of communication. The relationship with patients and families may extend over years or decades, in contrast to abbreviated hospital stays that are commonly seen in the era of managed care. The provider has an opportunity to have a breadth of knowledge about both an individual and dynamics that are occurring in their family and world. The clinician may have the chance to see families progress through many stages of development, experiencing both successes and losses.

In primary care, the patient sets the agenda by making the initial appointment and presenting the initial complaint with, at times, a limited ability to communicate their concern. In this setting the patient is free to disregard the opinion of the provider, and may seek the opinion of someone else in the practice or another practice clinician. According to Hewitt (1996), the majority of diagnoses can be made from history alone, about 5% of diagnoses can be decided by adding a physical examination, and only 1 to 2% require further investigation. These figures further highlight the importance of the ability to listen on the part of the provider.

Due to the long-term nature of many patient relationships the clinician can, over time, catch any changes that the patient presents, in terms of attitude, affect, and presentation. It may only be over time that a clinician could assess that a poorly groomed patient may be struggling with depression, based on the fact that they had, in the past, paid careful attention to grooming. If the patient seems to lack motivation to follow a particular treatment regime it is important to note if this is different from past presentation.

It is over time that relationships, of any kind, mature and deepen. Trust is initially developed and then, ideally, matures with repeated experiences between patient and provider. When the relationship has a stable foundation, providers gain the ability to broach difficult topics because their motivation is not called into question by the patient or family. The art of intervention informs the clinician in regard to the timing of communications that are difficult, but they are also informed by the strength of the relationship with the patient. Primary care offers the opportunity to develop lasting and deeply satisfying nurse–patient relationships.

The Family Connection

It is in primary care that a provider can also interface with the extended family of a patient. The family may accompany the patient only as far as the waiting room or into the patient room. Relationships with family members may also span over years or decades. Managing these relationships will test issues of confidentiality. This is particularly true if the patient is underage, and this issue is covered in the chapter on treating children and adolescents, Chapter 5. A growing area, however, is that of treating elders who may be living with adult children.

These family relationships may be complicated and the provider will do well to avoid making assumptions about these relationships, and may choose to see the elder alone at times in order to gain an accurate view of how they are experiencing their illness or life in general. Permission to share medical information is needed unless a guardian has been appointed.

Primary care is one of the few settings that allow relationships with patients and families to evolve over years and to mature. Providers may become very important people in the patient's life. The typical primary care visit may only last a matter of minutes, but the extended life of the relationship puts the relationship in a special category. The influence that a provider can have in regard to healthcare decisions can be significant. I know of a mother of an adolescent who had been trying to convince her daughter to submit to the series of immunizations for human papilloma virus (HPV) to no avail. After going to her primary care provider, for the benign issue of wart removal, the teen came home and announced that her primary care provider had recommended the immunization and she readily agreed and had, in fact, received the first of three injections during her office visit. The potency of the therapeutic relationship with the provider won the day and the conflict between mother and daughter was brought to an end.

Respect

Beach, Wang, Duggan, and Cooper (2006) studied the issue of *physician reported respect* for patients, patient's perceptions of physician respect, and whether specific communication behaviors could be correlated with respect. Results of the study include a positive correlation of familiarity and respect rather than sociodemographic variables—the fact that patients can correctly assess when they are respected and often overestimate physician respect. There was also a positive correlation between feelings of respect by physicians and provision of more information to patients.

It seems that patient *expectations* of how long a visit will be have an impact on patient satisfaction. Patients who assessed that their visit exceeded what they expected had higher levels of satisfaction and the reverse was also true (Lin et al., 2001). Health concerns and self-perceived health status were correlated with expectations for longer clinical visits. While the primary care physicians felt "rushed" 10% of the time, patients reported they thought the clinician was so in only 3% of the visits. Physicians estimated that patient satisfaction was lower when they felt rushed, but this was not born out by patient resorts. It was the expectation of time for the visit that was most related to patient satisfaction. A systematic review of randomized clinical trials and analytic studies of physician–patient communication confirmed a positive influence of quality communication on health outcomes (Stewart et al., 2000; Teutsch, 2003). Heritage, Robinson, Elliott, Beckett, and Wilkes (2007) tested out a method of assuring that all patients had the opportunity to get their needs met during a clinical visit. Simply by asking, "Is there anything else you want to address in the visit today?" and "Is there something else you want to address in the visit today?" the researchers found that patient's unmet concerns could be reduced by almost 80%.

In one study of effective methods of terminating a clinical visit, it was found that giving the patient a printed document was perceived as ending the visit, as well as verbal positive comments, such as "Be well" (Bronshtein, Katz, Freud, & Peleg, 2006). An interesting study of how physicians and patients communicate during the closing of office visits found that patients communicated new concerns 21% of the time (White & Roter, 1994) and the authors suggest that informing patients about the "flow of the visit," attending to assessing patient beliefs, and addressing psychosocial issues *early* in the visit can avoid difficulties at the end.

COMPLIANCE, ADHERENCE, AND FOLLOW-THROUGH

The notion of having a patient follow treatment recommendations is referred to as *compliance, adherence,* or *concordance.* The terms are often used interchangeably and often in the negative, such as noncompliance, nonadherence, or nonconcordance. It has become popular of late to use the term adherence, because to comply infers paternalism and a measure of submission on the part of the patient. Regardless of the term, all clinicians grapple with the issue of having patients actually take a prescribed medication or continue to monitor blood sugar or blood pressure, all in the name of patient adherence. The term nonadherence has replaced the former term of noncompliance even though they refer to same phenomenon—that of patients not following through on prescribed treatments of the healthcare provider.

In a meta-analysis reviewing over 1000 articles on the subject (DiMatteo, 2004) that reviewed predictors and outcomes related to adherence to chronic illness regimes, the author concluded that improvements in health professional–patient communications were the key to improved adherence. In regard to patient participation in medical encounters, research indicates that the strongest predictors are situation-specific, such as clinical setting and the physician's communicative style (Street, Gordon, Ward, Krupat, & Kravitz, 2005; Zandbelt, Oort, Godfried, & de Haes, 2007). In particular, supportive communication and partnership building were identified as being effective. Collaborative models of patient care have been studied and found to improve adherence (Funnell & Anderson, 2004; Kaplan & Frosch, 2005; Langford, Sawyer, Gioimo, Brownson, & O'Toole, 2007).

Improving Patient Compliance

Provider response to patients not making recommended changes in lifestyle or taking prescribed medications may include a feeling of loss of control regarding patient outcomes, confusion, anger, and frustration about patient behaviors. In addition, feeling detached from the patient can be a result of these feelings and these feelings can be generalized when dealing with other patients in ones' practice. Church (2000) suggests, rather than viewing adherence in the traditional manner, that clinicians reframe the issue and recognize the positive aspects of noncompliance, such as an opportunity to learn the natural course of disease, develop respect for patient autonomy, and learn more about patient motivation. The author reminds providers that, for some patients, "noncompliance a way to assert control" and, instead of focusing on what the patient is *not* doing, it is an opportunity to dialogue about what they want to do. This perspective places an emphasis on patient choice and empowerment and directly addresses the issue of the patient having control over their health. A plan becomes the patient's plan, instead of one imposed on the patient. During follow-up, if a patient-devised plan fails, then alternative plans can be devised, including the original ideas of the healthcare provider. By viewing noncompliance as an opportunity, the clinician may garner information into the patient's belief system and motivation. Church's (2000) suggestions for improving compliance are in Box 4-1.

Instead of experiencing noncompliance as a power struggle, it can be viewed as entry into discussing what might be getting in the way of following recommendations provided by the clinician. The conversation can switch from a scolding to an inquiry. "What got in the way of _____?" can reap interesting information if the clinician can manage to approach the patient in a nonjudgmental manner. Instead of assuming one knows why the patient did not follow through with recommendations, it is wise to ask. Any number of possible reasons may surface, including financial constraint, knowledge deficits, or cultural issues. Additional reasons for noncompliance may include patient fear regarding side effects, lack of information regarding medications or dosages, inconvenience, or psychological issues such as denial. The reasons may vary according to age groups as well. Elderly patients are often prescribed a myriad of medications and patients may struggle with issues related to memory. Middle-aged patients may be juggling a busy life and find it hard to take prescribed medications on time, or at all. Adolescents may act out their predictable struggle with autonomy by refusing to adhere to recommended treatments. While a provider can assume any of these to be true, it is important to seek the individual explanation from the patient themselves, if they are aware of what is behind their difficulty to follow a treatment plan. Before suggesting a pill box, examine with your patient what exactly is the obstacle for them. Do not assume it is laziness or a lack of valuing health, although these may sometimes be present. Once you provide a rationale for treatment recommendations you need to listen to the patient's perspective if these recommendations are not followed. It is important to not personalize a patient's

Box 4-1　Suggestions for Improving Compliance

Optimize access to care
Emphasize patient education
Use patient-centered communication during visits
Encourage patients to bring family and others in support system to appointments
Schedule regular follow-up visits
Specifically ask patients questions about potential treatment side effects
Choose less frequent dosing for medications (or other treatments) when possible
Offer less expensive alternatives (even if suboptimal) when cost is a critical barrier
Confirm data; ask patients to routinely bring in medication bottles, blood pressure logs, diaries; call pharmacies to check refills of prescriptions; check serum drugs levels, etc.
Implement mail or telephone reminder systems
Structure the environment (work schedule, visual cues, etc.) to facilitate compliance
Initially simplify treatment regimens and advance the complexity after the patient gains experience and buy in
Explore patient reasons in event of noncompliance
Obtain patient feedback to confirm patient understanding
Use team approaches in organizing delivery of healthcare services
Use interpreter and community leaders as cultural brokers
Create or creatively tap into community resources

lack of follow through. Although it may be related to the provider–patient relationship, there are also many other reasons for noncompliance. The goal is to ask your patient, explore the possible reasons, and work with them without feeling resentful, irritated, or jaded.

In an attempt to collaborate with patients, the American College of Physicians (ACP) has developed a series of *Health Tips*, which are a series of flash cards for patients about various chronic diseases, including post-heart attack care, chronic obstructive pulmonary disease (COPD), dementia, diabetes, flu, HIV/AIDS, hypertension, pain, peripheral artery disease, restless leg syndrome, depression, high cholesterol, osteoporosis, prostate cancer screening, and smoking. These flash cards, which are available for download, guide patients to ask both their primary care providers and pharmacists specific questions related to medications and overall care. These double-sided cards, written below the fifth-grade level and available in both English and Spanish, can be obtained at the ACP Web site at http://foundation.acponline.org/hl/htips.

When reviewing the vast literature on patient compliance or adherence, the importance of the patient–provider relationship is clearly represented. Effective clinician communication is linked to positive patient outcomes (Safran et al., 1998; Stewart, 1995). Clinical suggestion regarding lifestyle habits is associated with increased effort on the part of patients to change (Galuska, Serdula, & Ford, 1999; Kreuter & Bull, 2000; O'Connor, Prochaska, Pronk, & Boyle, 2001). This type of provider–patient dialogue requires the clinician to actively listen to the patient's questions and resistances to treatment recommendations. It calls for collaborative approaches, which level the power dynamics of the patient–provider relationship, in order for the patient to take an active role in their own health and health-related behavioral choices.

The use of contracts, both written and verbal, between patients and providers to address the issue of treatment adherence has been reviewed as it relates to patients with substance abuse, hypertension, and obesity (Bosch-Capblanch, Abba, Prictor, & Garner, 2007). While the results were mixed, there does seem to be evidence that contracts can assist in achieving increased patient satisfaction and patient participation. Another interesting intervention aimed at increasing patient adherence is that of providing a record of the clinical visit for patients. In a review of facial expressivity, smiling, eye contact, head nodding, and hand gestures, postural positions trials with cancer patient consultations findings support the practice and cite data that recordings are useful and informative for patients and their family and friends (Pitkethly, MacGillivray, & Ryan, 2008). Interestingly, recordings did not make patients more anxious or depressed. Providing information to parents of children discharged from the hospital regarding continued care has been studied in order to determine the effectiveness of both verbal and written information (Johnson,

Sandford, & Tyndall, 2008). Findings point to the efficacy of providing *both* verbal and written instructions to parents, as opposed to only verbal instructions. Berger, Coulehan, and Belling (2004) have examined the issue of the use of humor in patient interactions, which includes both risks and benefits.

NONVERBAL COMMUNICATION

Nonverbal communication includes communication that is devoid of words and includes eye contact, facial expression, body movements, and postures that convey a message. While there is not a great deal of research on the impact of nonverbal behavior during the clinical encounter, there is outcome evidence in the area of patient satisfaction. As one might imagine, physicians who are more nonverbally emotionally expressive are seen more positively by patients and are associated with greater patient satisfaction (Griffith, Wilson, Langer, & Haist, 2003). This may be related to the message that is given and received when the clinician makes eye contact with the patient or family. A more intimate relationship is implied along with a higher level of interest in the patient. Another area of nonverbal behavior studied within the patient–clinician interaction is that of an ability to accurately read patient cues of distress. The research suggests that success in this area is positively correlated with higher patient satisfaction, and a higher rate of patients keeping their office appointments (Roter, Frankel, Hall, & Sluyter, 2006).

COMMUNICATION EXERCISES

1. Initial Meeting

Pair off as patient and provider.

Patient:

You are a 45-year-old lawyer looking for a primary care provider and makes an appointment at the clinic.

Provider:

Develop an introductory statement regarding your professional credentials and your philosophy of patient care.
Switch roles.

Discussion:

How would you describe the provider's demeanor?

Was the provider hesitant, confident, clear?

As the patient, did you feel comfortable asking any questions? If so, why was that? If not, why not?

What suggestion might you provide to this clinician today?

Did the clinician ask you any questions? If so, what were they?

As the provider, analyze what it was like to explain yourself and your philosophy of care. What components need to be further developed? What components were well developed? What feedback did you receive from your partner? How will you change your initial presentation in future?

_____

_____

_____

_____

_____

_____

_____

_____

2. Active Listening

Pair off as patient and provider.

Patient:

State a fictitious health issue that you are struggling with (5 minutes).

Provider:

Repeat back to the patient their concern.

Discussion:

Was the provider description accurate? If not repeat your health issue again.

Patient:

Finish the sentence "I feel _____ about this concern."

Provider:

Repeat this in your own words.

Patient:

Complete this sentence: "I have contributed to this issue by _____."

Provider:

Repeat in your own words.

Discussion:

How accurate was your provider in repeating your feelings and your contribution?

Patient:

Complete this sentence: "What I would like to happen in regard to this is _____."

Provider:

Repeat in your own words.

Switch roles.

Discussion:

As the patient, what was this experience like for you? Give this feedback to your provider.

_____

_____

_____

_____

_____

_____

_____

_____

3. Eye Contact

Pair off as patient and provider.

Patient:

Share with your provider for 15 minutes the events of the past weekend's activities while *not* making any eye contact; then share again, this time keeping eye contact the entire time.

Discussion:

How did the two stories differ? How were you affected by the two stories?

What emotions arose in each story?

What thoughts occurred during each story?

Which style is more like your personal style of communication?

Switch roles and repeat.

Discussion:

Discuss what comes to mind when considering the topic of eye contact in a professional encounter. Is this different when dealing with certain types of patients? With colleagues? With those who supervise you? What is your usual style of maintaining eye contact in your personal life? What challenges exist for you?

_____

_____

_____

_____

_____

_____

_____

_____

4. Active Listening in Conflict

Pair off as patient and provider.

Patient:

Speak for 15 minutes describing a conflict in your life.

Provider:

Use skills of validation, clarification, and summation to display your understanding of this situation to the patient.

Discussion:

How long before your provider interrupted you?

How would you assess their skills at accurately portraying your conflict?

Did your provider seem invested in what you were saying? How was this demonstrated to you?

Describe your experience and provide feedback to your provider. What improvements might you suggest?

As the provider, how did you attempt to "actively" listen?

When did you interrupt? When were you tempted to interrupt?

What were you experiencing affectively while listening?

How did this experience match your personal style of being someone who listens?

Switch roles and repeat.

_____

_____

_____

_____

_____

_____

_____

5. Deception

Pair off as patient and provider.

Patient:

Tell a fabricated story about a past event, not necessarily a health concern, that is elaborate in detail and lasts for 5 minutes.

Provider:

Note eye movement and mannerisms that occurred during the telling of the story.

Switch roles and repeat.

_____

_____

_____

_____

_____

_____

_____

6. Summarizing

Pair off as patient and provider.

Patient:

Present a cluster of symptoms that are of concern to you. Provide a lengthy and complicated history of the problem. Express strong affect at various points, without naming the feeling. Be sure to correct the provider if they inaccurately summarize your story.

Provider:

Use summary statements that will summarize the patient's narrative. At times, purposely make a mistake to see if the patient will simply be compliant or will correct you.

Discussion:

Share the experiences of the patient and the provider. What was it like to have someone correctly and incorrectly hear your narrative? How did it feel as a provider to have a patient correct you? Did you find this easy or challenging?

Switch roles.

_____

_____

_____

_____

_____

_____

_____

_____

7. Summarizing

Pair off as patient and provider.

Patient:

You have been told that there is a concern with a routine colonoscopy and that further testing will be needed. You are frightened and yet are seeking information without having to tell your provider about your fears. You do not easily talk about feelings. You are not comfortable sharing feelings with others outside your immediate circle. When you tear up, you try and conceal it from the provider.

Provider:

Your patient has had abnormal findings on a routine colonoscopy and you are meeting to discuss further testing. Make use of therapeutic communication techniques which encourage the patient to open up to you. Make up of responses such as "Tell me more," "Go on," and other such prompts.

_____

_____

_____

_____

_____

_____

_____

_____

8. Reigning in the Overly Talkative Patient

Pair off as patient and provider.

Patient:

Overload the presenting complaint with at least three or four separate issues. Do not let the clinician get a word in before you launch into another topic. Speak rapidly and nonstop. Do not let any silences exist. Do not make eye contact, look only at your feet, and fidget throughout the interview.

Provider:

Respond to the patient attempting to organize the patient's concerns and keep the interview on track.

Discussion:

Share your experiences of the other
What was effective?

What was ineffective?

What suggestions do you both have for improvement?

_____

_____

_____

_____

_____

_____

_____

9. Body Language

Pair up with a peer.

The first person role plays experiencing the following:

> frustration
> embarrassment
> anxiety
> suspicious
> hostility

The second person must name what they think the first person is experiencing; after three attempts, the correct answer is provided.

Switch roles.

Discussion:

Discuss what cues were read correctly and which were misinterpreted. Exchange information regarding what you know about body language cues.

What body language was a dead giveaway?

_____

_____

_____

_____

_____

_____

_____

_____

10. Using "I" Statements

Pair up as narrator and listener. Take turns. One person relays a recent difficulty they had in a clinical situation with a patient or staff. Then relay the
same story *but* only using "I" statements.

The listener raises their hand every time the narrator does not use "I" when
relaying a situation.

Switch roles.

Discussion:

Discuss the challenges of using "I" rather than naming someone else in a
story. Did this get harder when the story was emotionally charged? How
many times did the narrator have to start their sentence over?

Discuss the effect on the listener of the two versions of the story.

What is the overall effect of using "I" in a conflictual or highly emotional
situation?

Practice using "I" statements for the next week, and report back to each
other at the conclusion of the week.

_____

_____

_____

_____

_____

_____

_____

_____

11. Labeling Patients

Pair off as two providers.

One provider begins the dialogue and uses pejorative terms to label a patient. Continue to pepper the conversation with labels about this patient or family.

The other provider responds to this conversation.

Discussion:

What feelings were generated in hearing a colleague label a patient in an unflattering way?

What was the method of response used?

What communication techniques could be utilized in this situation in future?

_____

_____

_____

_____

_____

_____

_____

_____

JOURNALING EXERCISES

1. Values Clarification

What values do you hold in regard to health?

What were the influences that contributed to the development of these values?

What are your values in regard to patient compliance?

Have you experienced in your clinical work a challenge to any of these values?

Describe these clinical situations.

What are your current unresolved value issues in regard to patient care, clinical practice, or role development as an advanced clinician?

_____

_____

_____

_____

_____

_____

_____

_____

2. Assessment of Communication Skills

How would you assess your skills as a communicator?

What are your particular strengths?

What areas need improvement?

Who most influenced you in your family as a communicator?

What type of patient situations do you find most difficult in regard to communication?

Address your comfort level with dealing with conflict.

Describe a difficult clinical encounter from the past week or month and explore why it was difficult. How can this clinical encounter go more smoothly in future? Share this entry with a peer.

_____

_____

_____

_____

_____

_____

_____

_____

3. Listening

Do you consider yourself a competent listener?

What information do you have to back up this assessment?

What are your strengths in regard to listening?

What are your limitations in regard to listening?

Who listens most to you in your life?

Who do you listen to most in your life?

What do you think are the gender issues related to listening?

What is the hardest part about listening to patients?

Write about a clinical encounter in which you disappointed yourself in your listening skills. Describe the patient and the setting. What interfered with your ability to listen? What ideas do you have today about how to respond differently to this patient or family?

Recall an encounter when you feel you effectively used listening skills.

_____

_____

_____

_____

_____

_____

_____

_____

4. Technical Skills and Communication Skills

How would you compare your technical and procedural skills in a clinical setting as opposed to your communication skills?

What is the tension between the two skills?

In your graduate training, has there been an emphasis on one skill over the other?

What are the informal messages you have received in your clinical training in regard to the importance of patient communication?

What have you observed in the clinical area regarding peers or other clinicians and patient communication?

What priority do you assign to therapeutic communication with patients in a clinical encounter?

Has this opinion changed over time?

Are you more comfortable with the history taking or physical examination portion of a clinical visit?

What are the obstacles to therapeutic communication in a clinical encounter?

_____

_____

_____

_____

_____

_____

_____

_____

5. Clinical Setting and Communication

Describe a clinical setting in which you are currently involved. Do you consider this a setting that is conducive to therapeutic communication? Why or why not?

What do you consider the ideal setting?

Who are the role models for therapeutic communication in this setting?

What are the organizational realities that impact this issue?

Who are the change agents in this setting?

Do these change agents value therapeutic communication?

What suggestions do you have for facilitating therapeutic communication in this setting?

_____

_____

_____

_____

_____

_____

_____

_____

6. Facilitating Communication Skills

What nonverbal behavior could a clinician utilize to enhance therapeutic communication?

Do you typically convey a hurried or nonhurried manner in patient encounters?

What is your typical range of facial expressions when engaging in therapeutic communication with patients?

How do you typically encourage patients to elaborate their stories?

Do you utilize touch in clinical encounters? Do you have any questions or concerns in regard to the use of touch?

Do you typically practice these facilitative behaviors? Why or why not?

_____

_____

_____

_____

_____

_____

7. Acceptance

Which illnesses or presenting complaints might generate emotions that make acceptance of the patient difficult?

Write about a recent patient or family who challenged your ability to be nonjudgmental and accepting. Describe the clinical encounter with a focus on your acceptance.

Was the patient's attitude difficult to accept?

What are your associations to this behavior?

Did you adequately explore this behavior with the patient? If not, why not? Explore an alternative response on your part to the patient or family.

_____

_____

_____

_____

_____

_____

_____

_____

8. Establishing Trust

Do you consider yourself a person who easily trusts others or finds it hard to trust?

In regard to your ability to establish trust with a patient or family, how do you assess your skills?

What strategies do you employ in order to establish trust with a patient or family?

How do you know when you are effective?

Recall a clinical situation that required you to pay particular attention to the requirement of establishing trust. What were the specifics of the clinical encounter? What efforts on your part were most successful?

Now recall a clinical encounter in which you feel you were not successful in establishing trust with a patient or family.

How do you explain the difficulty of establishing trust with this patient?

What would you do differently with this type of patient in the future?

What particular types of patients challenge your ability to establish trust? Describe these patients.

What strategies might you employ in the future with such patients?

What obstacles stand in your way of effectiveness in this area?

_____

_____

_____

_____

_____

_____

_____

_____

9. Responsiveness

Recall a clinical encounter in which you were responsive to a subtle cue from a patient or family.

What was the indirect or incomplete message you responded to?

Was the cue a gesture, tone of voice, or hesitation on the part of the patient?

How exactly did you convey your responsiveness to the patient?

What "labeling" behavior and dialogue have you overheard in a clinical setting in regard to a patient?

What was your internal response to this behavior?

What was your external response?

How do you understand this type of behavior on the part of healthcare professionals?

Assess the propensity for labeling in your family of origin.

Write about a time when you found yourself labeling a patient or a family—be specific.

How do you understand this when reflecting on it?

_____

_____

_____

_____

_____

_____

_____

_____

10. Eye Contact

In your personal life, assess your use of eye contact when speaking to others.

Is this different if you are first introduced to someone, as opposed to a friend?

What is the use of eye contact practiced in your family? Observe this when you get together with your family the next time.

What does maintaining constant eye contact with another person *feel* like to you?

If uncomfortable, on any level, explore this a bit further.

Write about the meaning of maintaining eye contact for you.

What is your professional position about maintaining eye contact with patients and families?

Consciously focus on this for the next week in the clinic and record the results.

_____

_____

_____

_____

_____

_____

_____

_____

11. Experiment in Eye Contact

Conduct the following experiment and record the results.

Pick a public area where people are sitting for an extended period of time (bus, subway, restaurant). Lock eyes with another individual, and do not look away, no matter how long the interaction. Make sure you are the one who maintains the eye contact *until* the other person breaks the contact.

Explore how you felt during the encounter.

Did it feel aggressive at all?

How did you feel when the other person looked away?

What effect were you left with at the end of the experiment?

_____

_____

_____

_____

_____

_____

_____

_____

12. Overly Talkative

How would you assess your style of communication? Very talkative is at one end of a continuum and quiet is on the other end.

Assess your friends and family members' style in a similar manner.

What is it like for you to be with very talkative people?

What challenges does communicating with a highly talkative person pose for you?

How do you manage dealing with highly talkative people in your personal life?

What thoughts do you have about your ability to work with this type of patient in a clinical encounter?

_____

_____

_____

_____

_____

_____

_____

_____

13. Deception

Recall a situation in your clinical experiences when you thought a patient was trying to deceive you.

Write about your thoughts and feelings about the interaction as it was occurring.

How did you process this encounter, if at all?

What are your thoughts and feelings about the encounter over time?

Discuss any residual thoughts or feelings about this patient or family or a category of patients or families that has developed as a result of this encounter.

_____
_____
_____
_____
_____
_____
_____
_____

14. Statements

Conduct experiments in your personal life with using "I statements" when in conversation with friends and family for a 24-hour period of time (without disclosing to them what you are doing).

Write about the interactions.

Did you notice any difference in your usual dialogues?

What effect did using "I" statements have on the discussion?

How did you feel using this technique?

Now, transfer the experiment into a clinical setting and record the results.

_____
_____
_____
_____
_____
_____
_____

15. Repeating the Last Two Words

Conduct the following experiment and record the results.

In a conversation with a friend or family member, utilize the technique of repeating the last two words. Continue throughout the entire conversation using this skill.

Write about what the experience was like for you.

How did it change the interaction?

Assess how often you use this technique in your personal life.

Now transfer this experiment into the professional area and utilize the technique with a patient.

Write about the interaction.

Were there any difficulties you encountered using this technique?

What is your assessment of the effect in a therapeutic interaction with a patient or a family?

_____

_____

_____

_____

_____

_____

_____

_____

REFERENCES

Beach, C., Wang, N. Y., Duggan, P., & Cooper, L. A. (2006). Are physicians' attitudes of respect accurately perceived by patients and associated with more positive communication behaviors? *Patient Education and Counseling, 62*(3), 8.

Beck, R. D., Daughtridge, R.,& Sloane, P. F. (2002). Physician-patient communication in the primary care office: A systematic review. *The Journal of the American Board of Family Practice, 15*(1), 4.

Berger, J. T., Coulehan, J., & Belling, C. (2004). Humor in the physician-patient encounter. *Archives of Internal Medicine, 164,* 6.

Bosch-Capblanch, X., Abba, K., Prictor, M., & Garner, P. (2007). Contracts between patients and healthcare practitioners for improving patients' adherence to treatment, prevention and health promotion activities. *Cochrane Database of Systematic Reviews,* (2), CD004808.

Bronshtein, O., Katz, V., Freud, T., & Peleg, R. (2006). Techniques for terminating patient-physician encounters in primary care settings. *Israeli Medical Association Journal, 8*(4), 4.

Butterworth, T. (2004). Lend me your ears. *Nursing Standard, 19*(13), 16.

Church, L. (2000). Dilemmas in family medicine education. *Family Medicine, 32*(1), 2.

Clark, H. H., & Krych, M. A. (2004). Speaking while monitoring addressees for understanding. *Journal of Memory and Language, 50*(1), 62–81.

Coates, J. (1986). *Women, Men and Language.* New York: Longman Inc.

Coulehan, J. (2005). Viewpoint: Today's professionalism: Engaging the mind but not the heart. *Academic Medicine, 80*(10), 7.

DiMatteo, R. (2004, June). *Patient adherence: Lessons from five decades of research.* Paper presented at the meeting of Academy Health, San Diego, California.

Funnell, M. M., & Anderson, R. M. (2004). Empowerment and self-management of diabetes. *Clinical Diabetes, 22*, 5.

Galuska, D. A., Serdula, M. K., & Ford, E. S. (1999). Are health care professionals advising obese patients to lose weight? *Journal of American Medical Association, 16*(282), 157.

Glass, L. (1992). *He says, she says: Closing the communication gap between the sexes.* New York: The Putnam Berkeley Group.

Greer, J., & Halgin, R. (2006). Predictors of physician-patient agreement on symptom etiology in primary care. *Psychosomatic Medicine, 68*(2) 5.

Griffith, C. H., Wilson, J. F., Langer, S., & Haist, S. A. (2003). House staff nonverbal communication skills and standardized patient satisfaction. *Journal of General Internal Medicine, 18*, 170–174.

Haidet, P., & Paterniti, D. A. (2003). "Building" a history rather than "taking" one: A perspective on information sharing during the medical interview. *Archives of Internal Medicine, 163*, 7.

Heritage, J., Robinson, J. D., Elliott, M. N., Beckett, M., & Wilkes, M. (2007). Reducing patients' unmet concerns in primary care: The difference one word can make. *Journal of General Internal Medicine, 22*(10), 4.

Hewitt, A. (1996). Communications in the setting of primary care. In P. F. Myerscough & M. J. Ford (Eds.), *Talking to patients: Keys to good communication* (pp. 130–141). Oxford: Oxford Medical Publications.

Johnson, A., Sandford, J., & Tyndall, J. (2003). Written and verbal information versus verbal information only for patients being discharged from acute hospital settings to home. *Cochrane Database of Systematic Reviews,* (4), CD003716.

Kaplan, R. M., & Frosch, D. L. (2005). Decision making in medicine and health care. *Annual Review of Clinical Psychology, 1*, 5.

Kreuter, M., & Bull, F. (2000). How does physician advice influence patient behavior? *Archives of Family Medicine, 9*(5), 426–433.

Langewitz, W., Denz, M., Keller, A., Kiss, A., Rüttimann, S., & Wössmer, B. (2002). Spontaneous talking time at start of consultation in outpatient clinic: cohort study. *British Medical Journal, 325*, 2.

Langford, A., Sawyer, D., Gioimo, S., Brownson, C., & O'Toole, M. (2007). Patient-centered goal setting as a tool to improve diabetes self-management. *Diabetes Educator, 33*(supplement 6), 5.

Lin, C. T., Schilling, L. M., Cyran, E. M., Anderson, S. N., Ware, L., & Anderson, R. J. (2001). Is patients' perception of time spent with the physician a determinant of ambulatory patient satisfaction? *Archives of Internal Medicine, 161*(11), 6.

Marvel, M. K., Epstein, R. M., Flowers, K., & Beckman, H. B. (1999). Soliciting the patient's agenda: Have we improved? *Journal of the American Medical Association, 281*, 5.

Mauksch, L., Dugdale, D., Dodson, S., Epstein, R. (2008). Relationship, communication and efficiency in the medical encounter: Creating a clinical model from a literature review. *Archives of Internal Medicine, 168*, 1387–1395.

O'Connor, P. J., Prochaska, J.O., Pronk, N. P., & Boyle, R.G. (2001). Professional advice and readiness to change behavioral risk factors among members of a managed care organization. *American Journal of Managed Care, 7*(2), 125–130.

Pitkethly, M., MacGillivray, S., & Ryan, R. (2008). Recordings or summaries of consultations for people with cancer. *Cochrane Database of Systematic Reviews,* (3), CD001539.

Rabinowitz, I., Tamir, A., & Reis, S. (2004). Length of patient's monologue, rate of completion, and relation to other components of the clinical encounter: observational intervention study in primary care. *British Medical Journal, 28*, 2.

Rao, J. K., Inui, T. S., & Frankel, R. M. (2007). Communication interventions make a difference in conversations between physicians and patients: A systematic review. *Medical Care, 45*(4), 10.

Reik, T. (1948). *Listening with the third ear.* New York: Farrar, Straus.

Rhoades, D. R., Finch, W. H., & Johnson, A. O. (2001). Speaking and interruptions in primary care office visits. *Family Medicine, 33*(7), 5.

Roter, D., Frankel, R., Hall, J., & Sluyter, D. (2006). The expression of emotion through nonverbal behavior in medical visits. *Journal of General Internal Medicine, 21*(S1), 7.

Safran, D.A., Taira, D. A., Rogers, W.H., Kosinski, M., Ware, J. E., & Tarlov, A. R. (1998). Linking primary care performance to outcomes of care. *Journal of Family Practice, 47*(2), 213–220.

Seaburn, D. B., McDaniel, S. H., Beckman, H. B., Silberman, J., & Epstein, R. M. (2005). Physician responses to ambiguous patient symptoms. *Journal of General Internal Medicine 20*(6), 2.

Stewart, M. A. (1995). Effective physician-patient communication and health outcomes: A review. *Canadian Medical Association Journal, 152*, 1423–1433.

Stewart, M. A., Brown, J. B., Donner, A., McWhinney, I. R., Oates, J., Weston, W., et al. (2000). The impact of patient-centered care on outcomes. *Journal of Family Practice, 49*(9), 9.

Street, R. L., Gordon, H. S., Ward, M. M., Krupat, E., & Kravitz, R. L. (2005). Patient participation in medical consultations: Why some patients are more involved than others. *Medical Care, 43*(10), 10.

Tannen, D. (1990). *You just don't understand.* New York: William Morrow and Company.

Teutsch, C. (2003). Patient-doctor communication. *Medical Clinics of North America, 87*(5), 31.

Urkin, J., Elhayany, A., Ben-Hemo, P., & Abdelgani, A. (2002). [Interruptions during consultations— harmful to both patients and physicians]. *Harefuah, 141*(4), 349–352.

White, J., & Roter, D. (1994). "Oh by the way": The closing moments of the medical visit. *Journal of General Internal Medicine, 9*(1), 5.

Zandbelt, L. C., Oort, F. J., Godfried, M. H., & de Haes, H. (2007). Patient participation in the medical specialist encounter: Does physicians' patient-centered communication matter? *Patient Education and Counseling, 65*(3), 7.

SUGGESTED READINGS

Buber, M. (1958). *I and thou* (R. G. Smith Trans.). New York: Charles Scribner's Sons.

Colliver, M. S., Willis, M. S, Robbs, R. S., Cohen, D. S., & Swartz, M. H. (1998). Assessment of empathy in a standardized-patient examination. *Teaching and Learning in Medicine, 10*, 8–10.

Delamater, A. M. (2006). Improving patient adherence. *Clinical Diabetes, 24*, 8.

Faucett, J. (2005). Peplau's theory of interpersonal relations. In J. Faucett (Ed.), *Contemporary nursing knowledge.* Philadelphia: F.A. Davis.

Fenichel, O. (1945). *The psychoanalytic theory of neurosis.* New York: W. W. Norton.

Fromm, E. (1956). *The art of loving.* New York: Harper & Row.

Fromm-Reichman, F. (1950). *Principles of intensive psychotherapy.* Chicago: University of Chicago Press.

Hojat, M. (2007). *Empathy in patient care.* New York: Springer Publishing Co.

Makoul, G., & Strauss, A. (2003). Building therapeutic relationships during patient visits. *Journal of General Internal Medicine, 18*(Suppl. 1), 275.

Mercer, S. W., & Reynolds, W. J. (2002). Empathy and quality of care. *British Journal of General Practice, 52,* 9–12.

Miller, P., & Eisenberg, N. (1988). The relation between empathy and aggressive and externalizing/antisocial behavior. *Psychological Bulletin, 103,* 324–344.

Myerscough, P. (1996). *Talking with patients* (3rd ed.). Oxford: Oxford Medical Publications.

Olson, J. K. (1997). Nurse-expressed empathy, patient outcomes, and development of a middle-range theory. *Image- The Journal of Nursing Scholarship, 29,* 71–76.

Orlando, I. (1961). *The dynamic nurse-patient relationship.* New York: Putman.

Peplau, H. E. (1991). *Interpersonal relations in nursing: A conceptual framework of reference for psychodynamic nursing.* New York: Springer Publishing Co.

Peplau, H. E. (1997). Peplau's theory of interpersonal relations. *Science Quarterly, 10*(4), 162–167.

Rodgers, C. (1958). *The characteristics of a helping relationship.* Personnel and Guidance Journal 37(1) 6–16.

Rodgers, C. (1961). *On becoming a person.* Boston: Houghton Mifflin Company.

Sleath, B., Rubin, R. H., Campbell, W., Gwyther, L., & Clark, T. (2001). Physician-patient communication about over-the-counter medications. *Social Science and Medicine, 53*(3), 13.

Williams, C. (1989). Empathy and burnout in male and female helping professionals. *Research in Nursing & Health, 12,* 169–178.

CHAPTER 5

Communication
Across the Life Span

COMMUNICATING WITH CHILDREN
Valerie A. Hart

A technical report from the American Academy of Pediatrics notes that communication with patients is typically "trial and error" and suggests that pediatricians look to other professionals, including advanced practice nurses (APN), to lead the way and "assist in the provision and modeling of effective communication with children and families" (Levetown, 2008). The report goes on to discuss the ethical and moral imperatives of including a child in discussions about their health and illness, no matter how uncomfortable this may be in practice. While this may be rare (Dixon-Woods, Young, & Henley, 1999), encouraging children to participate in their own care seems to be laudable goal. This seems most obvious when subjective information is required, such as levels of pain or achieving the goal of being a true health partner.

When treating children we are really talking about working with both parents and a child. Therefore, both must be included in the healthcare dialogue. In a clinical visit it is natural to assume that there will be a certain amount of hesitation on the part of the child, even when they have been prepared ahead of time. Since the adult or parent will typically be providing part of the history and background for the situation, it is important to find ways to build a connection to them while not ignoring the presence of the child. Many parents will be emotionally upset when dealing with a sick child and may need both clear information and reassurance. After gaining a sense of the purpose of the clinical visit from the adult caring for the child, the clinician needs to address the patient, the child. Relating at eye level can be helpful to decrease the intimidation factor. Speaking in a calm and friendly, age-appropriate manner is required. Asking the child what their concerns are might reveal different concerns that are relevant. While younger children may be less adept at verbal communication, having materials for drawing handy can facilitate the child's ability to "tell" their concerns.

While there may be variability in regard to how much information parents desire, and their preference to be involved in decision-making for the care of their child, there is some evidence that clinicians do not always gauge parents' preferences correctly. In one study, two thirds of nurses misjudged parents' communication preferences; half underestimated the information that parents wanted (Sobo, 2004). A systematic Cochrane Review of interventions, studied for a 5-year period beginning in 2001, found that evidence exists that both children and adolescents with cancer benefit from support, informational sessions, and interventions aimed at reintegration into school and social activities (Ranmal, Prictor, & Scott, 2008).

Many childhood illnesses will present as no real danger for the patient, but will cause much distress for parents. Providing background information and putting the condition in a context that the parent can understand is key. Parents will be concerned about the seriousness of a condition, the cause, and the course of illness and treatment. It is important to acknowledge the distress, even if it seems unwarranted. Be careful not to dismiss the concerns of a parent. As a clinician, you may have an understanding of the continuum of illnesses and frequency of presentation in your office. The parent may never have experienced this condition before and may have no frame of reference in terms of what sort of threat it poses for their child. Being able to provide information in a clear manner, devoid of jargon, that the parent can understand is the skill that is required. The clinician's aim is to educate the parent, and this can only be accomplished once their initial fears have been addressed.

Forming a relationship to the child should be another goal for the clinical visit. Asking them about themselves, their interests, and activities can round out your understanding of them beyond the narrow reason they have presented to the clinic. In primary care settings there is the opportunity to develop long-term relationships with children and families. Part of the satisfaction of this setting is the chance to see families over time and develop meaningful relationships as children grow up. Professional relationships can grow and mature over time as well. It may be easy to overlook the child who is hesitant and shy in an initial visit and only focus on the parent. This does nothing, however, to establish the foundation of what may be a long-term relationship.

There may be situations when the clinician wishes to speak or examine the child without the presence of the parent. Of course this must be handled sensitively, but may be required if any type of abuse is suspected. Children will only be willing to disclose this information to a trusted clinician. Your experience of a child over time will provide clues in regard to behavior that seems to be unusual. Asking about how school life is going is often a window into their emotional life. For children, school is their work and so it is the environment where any emotional discomfort will be acted out or expressed. If a child has had a change in grades or has begun to experience disruptive behavior at school, there is reason to inquire about what may be troubling them. These conversations may be more successful when conducted in private, without a parent present. Logistically, it may make sense to have both parent and child in the room together initially, then ask the parent to step outside for a time, and then invite the parent back in the room once your assessment of the issues is complete.

When treating children there is a requirement to reassure, educate, and form relationships with both the adults/parents and the child.

The topic of suspected sexual abuse requires sensitivity and skill on the part of the clinician. The interview must be conducted in a safe setting with an unhurried interviewer. Establishing trust with the patient is paramount and the ability to listen without pressuring the child (Myerscough & Ford, 1996). A referral to experts in this field is always an option, but the duty to report suspicions of sexual or physical abuse are a matter of state law.

Street (1991) identifies three elements of physician–parent–child communication as:

Informativeness: health information provided by the clinician

Interpersonal sensitivity: affective behaviors that communicate interest on the part of the clinician

Partnership building: based on collaborating with the child and the parents, including sharing their concerns during the consultation

DIFFICULT CONVERSATIONS WITH CHILDREN

We have discussed in a previous chapter the guidelines for delivering bad news to patients. In addition to paying attention to the environment, issues of conveying information and responding to the patient, there is evidence that the emotional response of the provider is a helpful aspect of the dialogue that facilitates a connection with the provider for the family (Chisholm, Pappas, & Sharp, 1997; Krahn, Hallum, & Kime, 1993). There may be a sense of urgency on the part of the family of a child who has received a serious diagnosis, such as cancer. Clinicians need to be sensitive to this reality when scheduling meetings that share laboratory or biopsy results. The family should be allowed to include whoever they wish at the meeting. The issue of including the identified patient requires judgment and discussion ahead of time. It may seem prudent to include the patient, especially if they are adolescent (Mack & Grier, 2004), to avoid the possibility of fantasy about what the true diagnosis or prognosis and to encourage the adolescent to be an active part of their treatment from the

Box 5-1   Guidelines for Having End-of-Life Conversations with Ill Children

Establishing an agreement regarding open communication between all caregivers and the patient and family. This agreement concerns what information is to be shared with whom, which will head off the possibility of misunderstandings at a later time.
Engaging the patient.
Exploring what the child knows and wants to know about their illness.
Explaining medical information, paying attention to the developmental level of the patient.
Empathize with the child's responses.
Encourage the child while avoiding false reassurance.

beginning. There is evidence that children want to receive information about their illness and treatment plan, and Beale, Baile, and Aaron (2005) have developed a guideline for end-of-life conversations with patients and families when the patient is a child or adolescent—the six Es are in Box 5-1.

These authors emphasize the fact that serious illness represents a loss of control and patients may be carried away by fantasy if they do not receive accurate information. They argue that providers of care to children who have serious and terminal illnesses are obligated to enter into discussions that allow the patients and families to voice their concerns. While these may be stressful interactions for providers, the benefit of having them far outweigh a tendency for avoidance. Providers need to develop strategies for managing the stressful realities of their career. These may include joining a peer group, journaling practice, and developing methods of debriefing emotionally difficult sessions.

COMMUNICATING WITH ADOLESCENTS

Adolescence is a time for experimentation and engaging in risky behavior, which presents specific challenges to clinicians working with teens. The issues most commonly treated when working with adolescents include pregnancy, sexually transmitted diseases, substance abuse, depression, as well as managing chronic illnesses such as type I diabetes. In addition, clinicians need to be on the lookout for disturbing clues regarding date rape and violence, substance abuse, and eating disorders (Scheiman & Zeoli, 2003).

There is an inherent tension between providing health care to this population in regard to confidentiality. Studies have shown that being willing to seek care with confidentiality is very important to adolescents (Cheng, Savageau, Sattler, & DeWitt, 1993; Thrall et al., 2000). The American Academy of Pediatrics, American Medical Association, and American Association of Family Physicians all have taken the position that attempts need to be made to increase available and confidential health care for adolescents. The passage of the Health Information Portability and Accountability Act (HIPAA) places additional pressures on the clinician to meet regulations while building a therapeutic relationship with patients. Prior to HIPAA, individual state laws defined confidentiality of health information and, therefore, protection varied. With HIPAA the federal regulation requires a standard of confidentiality for patients. In addition to state and federal regulations, most clinics have privacy policies when treating adolescents. When dealing with sensitive areas, such as sexual activity, these policies may not be comfortable for all parents and education has proven to be an effective intervention when this situation occurs (Hutchinson & Stafford, 2005). Parents typically understand the concept of a teen meeting alone with a clinician during a healthcare visit and it is clear that adolescents are more willing to communicate and receive health care when confidentiality is assured (Ford, Millstein, Halpern-Felsher, & Irwin Jr., 1997). It is wise for clinics and practices to develop a confidentiality statement that explains both legal and ethical limitations while attempting to maintain the therapeutic patient relationship. It is certainly advisable to have an alliance with parents; parents can work with the clinician in respecting the developing process of independence in their teen. The balancing act of relating to *both* parent and patient becomes even more delicate when treating the adolescent. This is because the patient may be in the process of attempting to individuate and separate from their parents and yet parents may be very involved in issues of their health. The clinician must walk the tightrope of establishing and maintaining a relationship with both parties. The most critical issue to navigate is that of privacy while establishing a trusting relationship with an adolescent. It is wise to follow the practice of seeing parent and adolescent together. Adolescents will be suspicious of side conversations that do not include them. It is important that they hear the concerns of their parents, and it is also vital that they have an opportunity to respond to the clinician with their concerns. Adolescence is a time of keeping secrets. How many of us told all to our parents? Clinicians need to provide the opportunity for talking privately with adolescents during a clinical visit. Concerns about sexual activity, drug and alcohol use, and other risky behavior are common during adolescence. Your adolescent patient may need information related to health behaviors and may need to discuss sensitive topics. Any patient's ability to broach a difficult topic will rely on the relationship with the provider. This is especially true with the adolescent population. Part of what makes working with this patient category so challenging is the fact that adolescents tend not to be very verbal, and the fact that they feel invincible.

It explains why adolescents engage in such risky behavior when they know it is hazardous. The defense mechanism of denial seems to insulate adolescents from fully feeling the anxiety related to taking risks with their health and their lives. The therapeutic relationship can be the factor that allows conversations about the importance of safe sex, designated drivers, and human papillomavirus (HPV) vaccinations to occur. Hall, Holmqvist, and Sherry (2004) stress the importance of understanding the perspective of an adolescent patient, paying attention to the interpersonal context of risk communication, and remaining respectful of the patient's autonomy when discussing sexual behavior. Maintaining a nonjudgmental attitude is critical during discussions of sexual behavior with any patient, but teens may be particularly concerned about a provider's disapproving attitude.

While relating to the adolescent, the clinician must be cognizant of the values of the parents. If they are in conflict with the desires or behaviors of the adolescent, the clinician needs to negotiate the divide. If there has been an ongoing relationship with the clinician, they may have additional status as the expert who really knows the adolescent.

In a review of communication strategies when working with children and adolescents about a family member's cancer diagnosis and treatment (Scott, Harmsen, Prictor, Sowden, & Watt, 2003), several conclusions were reached utilizing five different studies, both randomized and nonrandomized. The authors concluded that there is evidence to support group-structured interventions which may be useful in providing information to children and adolescents as well as improving "coping, anxiety, adjustment and wellbeing." Another innovative intervention is the use of email with adolescents. Email has proven to be a valuable adjunct to office visits with teens (Harvey et al., 2008). Adolescents are able to articulate their health concerns electronically even when they were unable to do so during a visit to a healthcare provider. It would seem that advanced practice clinicians need to be comfortable with this method of communication and find a systematic way to incorporate email into an overall strategy when working with adolescents.

COMMUNICATING WITH OLDER ADULTS
L. Susan Yetter

Effective communication is the cornerstone of a therapeutic relationship between an APN and a client. Quite simply, without effective communication, nurses cannot meet the healthcare needs of their patients. Communicating with older adults is often perceived as particularly challenging. Older adults often suffer from complex, chronic illnesses that may impact their abilities to understand necessary, complicated, healthcare information and interventions. The purpose of this section is to discuss the common communication issues with older adults, the impact of these issues on the well-being of older adults, therapeutic communication skills that may be used to overcome these issues, and using therapeutic communication skills to discuss difficult topics. Finally, the chapter concludes with communication and journaling exercises to demonstrate how to use these skills effectively.

THE USE OF ELDERSPEAK

Too often, communication with older adults is characterized by what Hummert has termed "elderspeak" (Hummert, 1994; Williams, Kemper, & Hummert, 2005). Elderspeak is a patronizing, overaccommodation speech pattern used to communicate with people who are thought to be less able to understand direct communication (Ryan, Bourhis, & Knops, 1991; Williams et al., 2005). Elderspeak is sometimes referred to as "baby talk" as it is characterized by simplified vocabulary and grammar, exaggerated intonation, higher pitch, and increased volume. This type of speech pattern is also characterized by shorter sentences and close-ended questions. Repetition is common. Often, diminutives such as "sweetie," "honey," and "dearie," are used as is the use of inappropriate pronouns ("How are *we* today, Mr. Jones? It is time for *our* bath?"). Frequently, tag questions are used ("You would like eggs for breakfast, wouldn't you?") instead of direct questions ("What would you like for breakfast?") (Williams et al., 2005).

Elderspeak is often used because of the pervasive stereotype that aging is consistently associated with a decline in comprehension and memory (Murphy, Daneman, & Schneider, 2006). As Giordano (2000) points out, there are natural changes associated with aging that make communication with older adults more challenging. During the aging process, there are perceptual changes in the sensory system as exhibited by a decline in vision and hearing. Often, these perceptual changes cause an older adult to lose details when communicating, and repetition is necessary. Aging may also cause difficulties in managing cognitive interference; in other words, there may be a decreased ability to ignore extraneous, irrelevant information such as noise or other conversations in the same room. Aging can cause a decrease in the speed in which we retrieve information and respond to situations (Giordano, 2000); therefore, response time in communication may be delayed. These natural changes in aging, however, do not necessarily correspond with the loss of comprehending and remembering information. All older people are not hard of hearing, less competent, or more forgetful (Williams et al., 2005). Unfortunately, younger healthcare providers who interact with older adults often assume the worst—that older adults are more forgetful, slower, more dependent, and less active. These stereotypes often lead to relationships with older adults that demonstrate an imbalance of power, control, and authority—relationships that may have dangerous consequences (Ryan et al., 1991).

The Impact of Elderspeak

Obviously, elderspeak is not an effective communication because it can easily cause misunderstanding, client dissatisfaction, and the poor exchange of information between an APN and a client. This poor communication could lead to medical problems and poor health quality (Ryan et al., 1991). Furthermore, older adults who experience elderspeak from healthcare provider may respond with dependent behavior, lower self-esteem, frustration, and little respect for the healthcare provider. Older adults experiencing elderspeak may respond in conversations with answers they believe the provider wants to hear, and not the truth. Today's older adults grew up regarding healthcare providers as omnipotent and may therefore feel disrespectful, disagreeing, or even speaking directly to a provider. As a result, older adults already at risk for isolation may ultimately become an uninvolved observer in their own health care (Edwards & Chapman, 2004).

Communication plays a significant role in establishing a relationship with a client; good relationships with clients are key to maintaining and promoting quality health care and quality of life. Effective communication with a client signals that the healthcare provider values that client as a person (Edwards & Chapman, 2004). Effective communication is an attempt to emotionally connect; the use of elderspeak with older adults may in fact have the opposite effect, alienating clients (Carpiac-Claver & Levy-Storms, 2007). Elderspeak can be easily perceived as demeaning and patronizing, implying client incompetence. Furthermore, the use of diminutives such as sweetie, may be interpreted as inappropriate intimacy. In addition to negatively affecting the relationship between the provider and the client, these perceptions and interpretations may actually precipitate a health decline in older adults, causing lower self-esteem, withdrawal, and isolation (Williams et al., 2005). Like anyone, older adults prefer communication that includes an "affirming emotional tone that balances care and control, communicating that the listener is competent to comprehend the message and to act independently" (Williams et al., 2005, p. 14).

HOW TO IMPROVE COMMUNICATIONS WITH OLDER ADULTS

The first step to improve communication with older adults is recognition by the healthcare provider that healthcare delivery will improve if communication improves. It is the provider's responsibility to facilitate the establishment of a quality relationship with the client. Developing a holistic point of view, in which the provider understands that it is the client who is expert about himself as a person, is vital. Getting to know the client as a person and asking such question as what is important to him or her, what are his or her expectations of life and health care, and what is his or her view of the world and life will help the provider recognize and understand the client as an individual. Each interaction with the client should be seen as an opportunity to improve the relationship and decrease the chances of miscommunication (Bethea & Balazs, 2007).

Effective communication is considerate and supportive without condescension. Effective communication between a provider and a client demonstrates that the provider is knowledgeable and caring and that the client is competent and independent. There is a balance of care and control, as each participant is able to freely express information and feels the other is truly hearing what is being said. Effective communication is, therefore, based on mutual respect and understanding (Ryan et al., 1991).

To begin effective communication with an older adult, the provider must first reserve judgment and allow the client to explain concerns at their own pace. It is important to allow the client to identify problems in their own words. The healthcare provider should be aware of environmental distractions, such as a noisy hallway or squeaky chair. Furthermore, the provider must pay attention to the client: looking directly at the client, writing or tapping on the computer keys as little as possible (Giordano, 2000). As information is exchanged, the provider should frequently ask for feedback to ensure the client understands. When discussing a technical procedure, asking the client to repeat back the details can help clarify any misunderstandings. Nodding the head and offering frequent verbal acknowledgement while using good eye contact will encourage the client to continue explaining concerns. It addition to acknowledgement, it is important to allow for periods of reflection so the client has time to process information and further answer questions if necessary (Giordano, 2000).

Speech should be clear and concise, without the use of medical jargon. Older adults with hearing deficits often hear lower pitched voices more easily, so using a deep, clear voice may be helpful (as opposed to the high pitch of elderspeak). Direct questions, such as "how many hours of sleep do you get each night?" are more helpful and respectful than "you're not having any trouble sleeping are you?" Interactions should be comprehensive and nondirective; like younger people, older adults do not want to be told what to do and would prefer being included in the decision-making process. Asking clients how they would prefer to treat their high blood pressure will be much more effective than telling them to take an antihypertensive medication or to lose weight. Discussions about medical interventions with older adults should be respectful, compassionate, and inclusive; the quality of health care provided is directly related to the tone and nature of these discussions.

Difficult Conversations with Older Adults

Conversations with older adults may not only be challenging because of communication styles, but also because discussions with older adults often focus on difficult issues, such as mistreatment and end-of-life care. The next section discusses approaches that may be helpful when broaching these topics with older adults.

ELDER MISTREATMENT

The role of the APN is often that of gatekeeper; it is the APN who assesses and treats clients on the "front lines" of primary care. Therefore, it is the APN who is ideally positioned to assess, treat, and refer victims of mistreatment. Assessment of mistreatment should be part of any routine exam and evaluation. The questions about mistreatment should be offered in a supportive, nonthreatening manner. Such questions that are posed with a nonjudgmental, matter-of-fact attitude will be more successful in discovering situations of abuse or mistreatment than questions posed with what may be perceived as a more critical attitude. Mistreatment of older adults is extremely difficult to detect because victims often feel embarrassed, intimidated, overwhelmed, and fearful of retaliation; the goal of any discussion is to prevent older adults from experiencing these feelings. Mistreatment of older adults encompasses physical, psychological, and sexual abuse; neglect and self-neglect; and financial exploitation. Physical abuse includes any sort of bodily injury, while psychological abuse includes verbal harassment, intimidation, and threats. Sexual abuse includes any form of intimate sexual activity without consent, including those who are unable to provide consent. Neglect can include the passive neglect from lack of information or resources, such as when care is provided to an older adult by someone who is mentally disabled or incompetent. Active neglect is malicious and includes neglect that is a result of disinterest or dislike. Self-neglect is defined as the inability to care for oneself, maintain safety, or manage financial issues (Wagner, Greenberg, & Capezuti, 2002). All types of neglect and abuse warrant investigation, intervention, and possible referral to state agencies. When dealing with a situation of mistreatment, it is imperative that the APN facilitate the assessment and resolution of mistreatment situations while respecting "patient autonomy and family sensitivities" (Carney, Kahan, & Paris, 2003, p. 73), so that the mistreatment is addressed without alienating the older adult and causing further family conflict and stress.

Asking questions when suspecting elder mistreatment is vital, and questions should be specific, direct, and explicit, while maintaining trust and rapport

(Acierno, Resnick, Kilpatrick, & Stark-Riemer, 2003). Often older adults fear placement in long-term care or assisted living, and would rather be mistreated in their own homes than move to a residential facility (Swagerty, Takahashi, & Evans, 1999). In addition to direct questions, it is important to note subtle or confusing complaints, inconsistencies, and vague or implausible explanations. It is also important to interview the older adult without the suspected abuser; if the suspected abuser refuses to leave, it is important to explore the reasons behind the refusal and make every attempt to interview the older adult and suspected abuser separately. Mistreatment of older adults is often the result of a stressed caregiver situation, so offering empathy, support, and community resources to the caregiver may be the key in stopping mistreatment and preventing further episodes in the future (Swagerty Jr. et al., 1999).

Interview questions about possible mistreatment start with general questions and progress to the specific. General questions would include: How do you and (*suspected abuser*) get along? Is (*suspected abuser*) treating you well? What happens when the two of you disagree? Do you need (eye glasses, hearing aid, false teeth, etc.)? How will you get those? How do you get help if you need it? More specific questions would include: Have you ever been threatened with punishment, deprivation, or institutionalization? Has anyone, including family members or friends, ever physically attacked you so that you have some degree of injury? Are you afraid of anyone? Have you ever been tied down or locked in a room? Are you alone a lot? Has anyone ever taken anything of yours without asking? Has anyone ever touched you or tried to touch you without your permission? Has anyone been insulting to you or using degrading language? Who pays the bills? Have you ever signed documents that you do not understand? Are any of your family members showing a great deal of interest in your money? (Acierno et al., 2003).

Questions for the suspected abuser should be similarly posed with respect. These questions would include: What is a typical day like? What support do you have? Do you ever get a break? Have you considered respite care? What are your expectations of the older adult? What care does the older adult require? Again, observe for inconsistencies, vague answers, and implausible explanations. All questions of the older adult and suspected abuser should be offered in a compassionate and professional manner, as this approach will glean more information than an accusatory approach. It is important to gather as much information without the suspected abuser becoming defensive and less likely to bring the older adult to appointments in the future (Wagner et al., 2002).

Obviously, these interview questions also usually accompany a physical exam, during which hygiene, cleanliness, appropriate dress, weight, skin turgor, skin appearance, and the presence of lesions, lacerations, hematomas, and other bodily injuries are particularly evaluated. If the injuries warrant, the mistreated older adult should be hospitalized. A referral to a visiting nurse service may be very helpful in getting a better picture of the home life and provide the older adult and caregiver with additional resources and support. If abuse and mistreatment are even remotely suspected, the APN is mandated to report the situation to state Adult Protective Services. Additionally, a referral to the Area Agency on Aging may provide linkage with community services, such as Meals on Wheels, respite care, and adult day care, which could ease caregiver burden. Finally, all information collected must be carefully and thoroughly documented in the medical record. The information should include a description of the situation, the medical and social history, the physical exam, including photos, and referrals made (Wagner et al., 2002).

As an advocate of the older adult, the APN's goal is to maintain the safety of the older adult. Using therapeutic communications skills to achieve this goal will maintain the sometimes tenuous trust and rapport established between an APN and the older adult client, and ultimately lead to high-quality nursing care of the client.

ADVANCED CARE PLANNING

Similar to assessing for mistreatment, discussion of advanced care planning should also be part of routine clinical care. It is the APN's responsibility to discuss with an older adult client what advanced care planning is, the importance of advanced care planning, and how to implement an advanced care plan. Discussing end-of-life care also requires compassion and respect. The APN must provide an environment in which dialogue about care options can occur openly and easily. The older adult client may require education about options for health care, including the benefits and burdens of different types of interventions. An older adult may be clear that they do not want "to be kept alive by machines," but often decisions about specific interventions such as ventilators, tube feedings, and intravenous (IV) fluids and antibiotics require education and clarification about potential end-of-life situations, treatment options, and treatment implications (Tuch & Strumpf, 2002).

It is the responsibility of the APN to first explore with the older adult what sort of goals for care are desired. Does the older adult want comfort measures only? Does the client want all possible medical interventions? Is the goal of care curative or palliative? What sorts of interventions are provided with these goals? The inconsistencies between the goals of care and the interventions that are wanted should be explored with the older adult. Furthermore, many of these explorations and discussions should occur with the older adult's family present (Smith, Davis, & Krakauer, 2007). After all, it is often the family members who make decisions in the last days of an older adult's life, and it is imperative that they be aware of the older adult's wishes. APNs must not only provide this information in a respectful and professional manner, but must also act as the older adult client's advocate. The role of advocate may require the APN to explain, educate, and clarify the desires and wishes of the older adult with the family repeatedly. The APN must recognize that these discussions can be stressful and difficult for everyone, especially family members, so the role of advocate also requires a calm, compassionate, and supportive demeanor.

In summary, communication with older adults should not be any different than communicating with other clients. Effective communication with older adults is based on respect and the recognition of the older client as a competent, independent individual with valid concerns. Effective communication with older adults is not only important in building a therapeutic relationship, but it is vital in providing quality health care.

Included at the end of the chapter are communication exercises that may be helpful in improving communication skills with older adults.

COMMUNICATION EXERCISES

1. Therapeutic Relationship

Pair off as provider and child: 30 minutes.

Provider:

Conduct an intake interview while attempting to form a bond with this patient.

Patient (child):

Present a challenging picture to the provider in regard to working with you.

Discussion:

How is an interview with a child different from working with an adult?

What were the strong components of the interview?

What were the limitations?

What lessons might be applicable next time you work with a child in a clinical encounter?

Switch places and repeat.

_____

_____

_____

_____

_____

_____

_____

_____

2. Working With a Teen

Work as a trio, as provider, teen, and parent: 60 minutes.

Provider:

Your adolescent patient presents in the examination room with a parent present. Take the interaction from there, dealing with both the patient and the parent.

Patient:

Pick a sexual issue for your concern, one you naturally feel uncomfortable talking about in the presence of your parent.

Discussion:

Debrief this interaction from all positions as provider, teen, and parent. **Switch roles until all have a chance to play all roles.**

_____

_____

_____

_____

_____

_____

_____

_____

3. Elderspeak

Pair off as provider and older adult patient. Props needed: sunglasses, cotton balls, petroleum jelly.

Provider:

Perform health history, taking into account the sensory deficits without using elderspeak.

Patient:

Wear the sunglasses with petroleum jelly on the lenses and place the cotton balls in your ears to simulate hearing and vision deficits.

Discussion:

What challenges did you encounter as the provider? As the client? How did you overcome the tendency to use elderspeak? How might this exercise help in encounters with actual older adults with sensory deficits?

Switch roles.

_____
_____
_____
_____
_____
_____
_____
_____

4. Observing Elderspeak

Visit a long-term care facility and observe the interactions between the staff and the residents. How would you describe their interactions? How often did you observe the use of elderspeak? How could the interactions occurred without the use of elderspeak? What challenges does the staff face in eliminating the use of elderspeak?

_____
_____
_____
_____
_____
_____
_____

5. Mistreatment

Pair off as provider and older adult patient.

Provider:

You suspect your older adult client is a victim of mistreatment. During the assessment, include questions about mistreatment.

Discussion:

As the APN, how difficult was it to ask these questions?

As the older adult client, how difficult was it to answer these questions?

What would make asking these questions easier?

JOURNAL EXERCISES

1. Communicating with Children

How would you assess your skills in communicating with children?

Describe your personal experience with children.

Identify difficult situations with this population.

Recall a recent clinical experience with a child and parent that was confusing or particularly difficult.

Describe the specifics of the clinical encounter.

What were the challenges in this encounter?

Was it more difficult dealing with the adult (parent) or the child? Explain why this was.

What communication techniques did you utilize which were effective?

What communication techniques did you utilize that were ineffective?

Why do you suppose this encounter was challenging?

How might you adjust your communication in similar clinical encounters in the future?

_____

_____

_____

_____

_____

_____

_____

_____

2. Communicating with Adolescents

Describe a recent clinical encounter with an adolescent patient that was challenging.

Was the parent present during the entire interview?

How did you instruct the patient and parent in regard to issues of confidentiality?

What made the clinical encounter challenging?

What are your personal experiences with adolescents?

Was your adolescence particularly stormy?

How does recalling your own adolescence inform your clinical skills with this population?

Is this a population that you enjoy or tolerate professionally?

What specific techniques can you think of that might have made this encounter more satisfying?

What might you do differently in future?

_____

_____

_____

_____

_____

_____

_____

_____

3. Confidentiality

After researching what the legal constraints regarding confidentiality with adolescents are in a practice setting, interview a clinician and report on what controversy exists in this area.

Share this with a peer and discuss.

_____

_____

_____

_____

_____

_____

_____

_____

4. Risky Health Behaviors

Write about yourself as an adolescent and identify any risky behaviors that you indulged in, including health-related behaviors.

Recall what you were thinking and feeling at the time.

How do you understand this behavior now?

If you have children of your own, how does it color your thoughts about risky behaviors?

How might thinking of these incidents affect your working with adolescents?

_____

_____

_____

_____

_____

_____

_____

_____

5. Email and Clinical Care

Pick a peer and play the parts of provider and teen patient.

Communicate via email after a clinical visit.

Discussion:

What is the value of email and clinical care?

What are the drawbacks of email and clinical care?

How comfortable are you with electronic communication in general?

Interview clinicians in a practice setting to get their thoughts on using email in clinical settings.

_____

_____

_____

_____

_____

_____

_____

_____

_____

6. Communicating with Older Adults

Discuss and describe your own experience with older adults.

What role did your grandparents play while you were growing up?

What was your experience with them?

What was your relationship with them or other older adults?

Reflect on how that relationship impacts your interactions with older adults today.

_____

_____

_____

_____

_____

_____

_____

_____

7. Elderspeak

Discuss and describe a relationship with an older adult that you have currently or have had in the past.

What type of relationship was it?

What role, if any, did elderspeak play?

How do you feel about that relationship?

How do you think the older adult regarded your relationship?

How does that relationship affect your current thoughts and attitudes about older adults?

When you encounter an older adult in the community, how do you interact with that person?

_____

_____

_____

_____

_____

_____

_____

_____

8. Mistreatment

Discuss your thoughts and feelings about the mistreatment of older adults.

How would you manage a situation of mistreatment as an APN?

What difficulties might you encounter, especially when assessing the suspected abuser?

Remembering that mistreatment may be the result of a stressful caregiving situation, how might you approach the suspected abuser?

_____

_____

_____

_____

_____

_____

_____

9. Advanced Care Planning

Discuss your thoughts and feelings about end-of-life care. What are your beliefs about medical interventions in the care of older adults? How might your beliefs affect your conversations about advanced care planning with older adult clients and their families?

_____

_____

_____

_____

_____

_____

_____

REFERENCES

Acierno, R., Resnick, H., Kilpatrick, D., & Stark-Riemer, W. (2003). Assessing elder victimization—demonstration of a methodology. *Social Psychiatry and Psychiatric Epidemiology, 38*(11), 644–653.

Beale, E. A., Baile, W. F., & Aaron, J. (2005). Silence is not golden: Communicating with children dying from cancer. *Journal of Clinical Oncology, 23*(15), 3629–3631.

Carney, M. T., Kahan, F. S., & Paris, B. E. (2003). Elder abuse: Is every bruise a sign of abuse? *The Mount Sinai Journal of Medicine, 70*(2), 69–74.

Carpiac-Claver, M., & Levy-Storms, L. (2007). In a manner of speaking: Communication between nurse aides and older adults in long term care settings. *Health Communication, 22*(1), 59–67.

Cheng, T. L., Savageau, J. A., Sattler, A. L., & DeWitt, T. G. (1993). Confidentiality in health care: A survey of knowledge, perceptions, and attitudes among high school students. *Journal of American Medical Association, 269*, 1404–1407.

Chisholm, C. A., Pappas, D. J., & Sharp, M. C. (1997). Communicating bad news. *Obstetrics and Gynecology, 90*(4), 637–639.

Dixon-Woods, M., Young, B., & Henley, D. (1999). Partnerships with children. *British Medical Journal, 319*, 778–780.

Edwards, H., & Chapman, H. (2004). Contemplating, caring, coping, conversing: A model for promoting mental wellness in later life. *Journal of Gerontological Nursing, 30*(5), 16–21.

Ford, C. A., Millstein, S. G., Halpern-Felsher, S. G., & Irwin Jr, C. E. (1997). Influence of physician confidentiality assurances on adolescents' willingness to disclose information and seek future health care. *Journal of American Medical Association, 278*(12), 1029–1034.

Giordano, J. A. (2000). Effective communication and counseling with older adults. *International Journal of Aging & Human Development, 51*(4), 315–324.

Hall, P. A., Holmqvist, M., & Sherry, S. B. (2004). Understanding and managing risky sexual behavior in adolescents. *Medscape Topics in Advanced Practice Nursing eJournal, 4*(1).

Harvey, K., Churchill, D., Crawford, P., Brown, B., Mullany, L., Macfarlane, A., & McPherson, A. (2008). Health communication and adolescents: What do their emails tell us? *Family Practice, 25*(4), 304–311.

Hummert, M. L. (1994). Stereotypes of the elderly and patronizing speech. In M. L. Hummert, J. M. Wiemann, & J. F. Nussbaum (Eds.), *Interpersonal communication in older adulthood* (pp. 162–185). Thousand Oaks, CA: Sage.

Hutchinson, J. W., & Stafford, E. M. (2005). Changing parental opinions about teen privacy through education. *Pediatrics, 116*(4), 966–971.

Krahn, G. L., Hallum, A., & Kime, C. (1993). Are there good ways to give "bad news"? *Pediatrics, 91*(3), 578–582.

Levetown, M. (2008). Communicating with children and families: From everyday interactions to skill in conveying distressing information. *Pediatrics, 121*(5), 1441–1460.

Mack, J. W., & Grier, H. E. (2004). The day one talk. *Journal of Clinical Oncology, 22*(3), 536–566.

Murphy, D. R., Daneman, M., & Schneider, B. A. (2006). Why do older adults have difficulty following conversations. *Psychology and Aging, 21*(1), 49–61.

Myerscough, P. R., & Ford, M. (1996). *Talking with patients: Keys to good communication.* New York: Oxford University Press.

Ranmal, R., Prictor, M., & Scott, J. T. (2008). Interventions for improving communication with children and adolescents about their cancer. *Cochrane Database of Systemic Reviews*, (4), CD002969.

Ryan, E. B., Bourhis, R. Y., & Knops, U. (1991). Evaluative perceptions of patronizing speech addressed to elders. *Psychology and Aging, 6*, 442–450.

Scheiman, L., & Zeoli, A. M. (2003). Adolescents' experiences of dating and intimate partner violence: "Once is not enough." *Journal of Midwifery & Women's Health, 48*(3), 226–228.

Scott, J. T., Harmsen, M., Prictor, M. J., Sowden, A. J., & Watt, I. (2003). Interventions for improving communication with children and adolescents about their cancer. *Cochrane Database of Systemic Review*, (3), CD002969.

Smith, A. K., Davis, R. B., & Krakauer, E. L. (2007). Differences in the quality of the patient-physician relationship among terminally ill African American and white patients: Impact on advance care planning and treatment preferences. *Journal of General Internal Medicine, 22*, 1579–1582.

Sobo, E. J. (2004). Good communication in pediatric cancer care: A culturally-informed research agenda. *Journal of Pediatric Oncology Nursing, 21*(3), 150–154.

Street, R. L. (1991). Information-giving in medical consultations: The influences of patients' communicative styles and personal characteristics. *Social Science and Medicine, 32*, 541–548.

Swagerty, D. L, Takahashi, P. Y., & Evans, J. M. (1999). Elder mistreatment. *American Family Physician, 59*(10), 2804–2808.

Thrall, J. S., McCloskey, L., Ettner, S. L., Rothman, E., Tighe, J. E., & Emans, S. J. (2000). Confidentiality and adolescents' use of provides for health information and for pelvic examinations. *Archives of Pediatrics and Adolescent Medicine, 154*, 885–892.

Tuch, H., & Strumpf, N. E. (2002). Palliative care. In V. T. Cotter, & N. E. Strumpf (Eds.), *Advanced practice nursing with older adults*. New York: McGraw-Hill.

Wagner, L., Greenberg, S., & Capezuti, E. (2002). Elder abuse and neglect. In V. T. Cotter, & N. E. Strumpf (Eds.), *Advance practice nursing with older adults: Clinical guidelines* (pp. 319–332). New York: McGraw-Hill.

Williams, K., Kemper, S., & Hummert, M. L. (2005). Enhancing communication with older adults: Overcoming elderspeak. *Journal of Psychosocial Nursing, 43*(5), 12–16.

CHAPTER 6

Difficult Conversations

Valerie A. Hart

COMMUNICATING BAD NEWS

Conceal most things from the patient while you are attending to him. Give necessary orders with cheerfulness and serenity . . . revealing nothing of the patient's future or present condition. For many patients . . . have taken a turn for the worse by forecast of what is to come.

—Hippocrates

The construct of delivering bad news conveys a construct of detachment and one-way communication on the part of the practitioner. Mail is delivered. Pizza is delivered. A frightening diagnosis or prognosis should never be delivered. It should be broached in the context of a relationship of mutuality and reciprocity.

—Browning, 2003

In the course of patient and family interactions there will occur the need to communicate "bad news" regarding a clinical condition. The news might involve information that is a surprise to the patient, or confirms their worst fear. Bad news may be defined as "any information which adversely and seriously affects an individual's view of his or her future" (Buckman, 1992, p. 15). There has occurred a clear shift in regard to informing patients about bad news, evidenced by Hippocrates's words. The medical community initially was concerned about protecting patients and families from bad news. Today, the topic falls into areas related to patient/family-centered care, informed consent, and legal and ethical clinical practice.

The majority of cancer patients desire detailed information concerning their illness, including prognosis data, and this information varies depending on the stage of the illness (Butow, Dowsett, & Hagerty, 2002; Derdiarian,1986; Glass & Douglas, 2004; Greisinger, Lorimore, & Aday, 1997; Jenkins, Fallowfield, & Saul, 2001; Leydon, Boulton, & Moynihan, 2000; Sapir, Catane, & Kaufman, 2000). Clinicians have both a legal and ethical responsibility to provide clear information so that patients and families can make informed decisions regarding care.

The literature reveals that communicating bad news is stressful for the clinician and may be more stressful for the inexperienced provider, when the patient is young, when the clinician and patient have a longstanding relationship, when strong optimism for a successful outcome had been previously expressed, and when the prospects for effective treatment are limited (Baile, 2000). A recent study found that oncologists infrequently responded with empathic responses even when opportunities presented themselves during a clinical visit (Pollak et al., 2007).

Clinicians find it hard to communicate bad news because of several factors, including a fear of being blamed, fear at unleashing a reaction, fear of expressing emotions, fear of not knowing all the answers, and fear of death (Buckman, 1992). Research supports the contention that oncology nurses lack sufficient training and feel ill prepared in the area of communication skills. Nurses report feeling most challenged when faced with patients dealing with death and dying and euthanasia requests (Sivesind et al., 2003). A lack of communication skills on the part of providers has been shown to lessen patient disclosure, cause anxiety for patients, and decrease satisfaction of care provided (Kennedy, 2005). Communication skills workshops for advanced practice nurses working with standardized oncology patients has proved to be effective and is recommended for inclusion early in the curriculum and reinforced throughout (Rosenzweig, Clifton, & Arnold, 2007). Various communication skills training workshops have proven results in the area of oncology (Fellowes, Wilkinson, & Moore, 2003; Razavi & Delvaux, 1997). Calling upon lessons learned in palliative care, Barnard (1995) speaks of the tension for providers between achieving moments of intimacy with patients and their own mortality and a fear of their own undoing. Facing this tension means acknowledging the spiritual nature of the tension—facing the reality that we are all finite human beings seeking meaning and love in the face of death who hope to face our own end with courage. These are the issues that are touched on when we interact with someone with a terminal illness, and that may press on us to avoid the conversation altogether. De Haes and Koedoot (2003) speak of the paradoxes of utilizing a patient-centered approach when working in palliative care where many patients want to avoid receiving information and making decisions, deferring to the clinician. In turn, clinicians may choose more aggressive therapies rather than "watchful waiting" in order to avoid painful discussions with patients. Patients may wish to remain hopeful and resist being fully informed regarding prognosis, and clinicians may collude rather than confront harsher realities that would lead to discussing supportive measures and end-of-life care. Less intrusive therapies may never be discussed while aiming to respect a patient's defenses.

While difficult news is best communicated within the context of an ongoing therapeutic relationship, the same principles of provider–patient relationships apply even if it is a one-time encounter.

In one study, cancer patients expressed a preference for their clinician to sit rather than stand when communicating bad news (Bruera et al., 2007). In addition, sitting physicians were rated as being more compassionate by patients. However, the research also found that sitting alone cannot compensate for poor communication skills or a lack of respect, in general, expressed during a clinical visit.

Cancer patients desire detailed information about their illness and, in addition, wish to receive the information about the illness as well as treatment options as soon as it is certain (Parker et al., 2001). In addition, female patients placed more importance on getting detailed information and receiving support from their caregiver. Patients with more formal education cited the context of how the news was given as being important than those with less education. These findings did not differ according to stages of cancer or whether the illness was a recurrence or not.

Barriers to communicating bad news include: denial on the part of the clinician; filtering the information by using jargon; fear of lessening the patient's hope; remaining emotionally distant; and leaving the treatment with the patient (Coulehan & Block, 2001). Studies reveal that if the clinician considers the bad news a defeat, it causes a delay in informing the patient, while more and more diagnostic tests are ordered. Clinicians may also use the classic defense mechanism of projection when stating, "I don't think the patient can handle the news." Projection is an unconscious process and, like all defense mechanisms, serves a protective function. Denial on the part of the provider will not serve the patient or family well. Depending on complicated medical explanations when delivering bad news is also a form of protection, as a clinician can seek refuge behind the comfort of jargon. It does nothing to fully inform the patient, however. Overly intellectual or complex descriptions or the use of vague terms may comfort the provider and confuse the patient or family. Being ambiguous is another form of communication that is obstructive when simple explanations and inquiries can be made. If hope is defined by the clinician as either curing a patient or bringing about remission, then a discussion of a terminal illness flies in the face of the caregiver's mission in regard to patient care. Neuland (1993) suggests that differentiating hope of cure must be abandoned in place of human hope. Clinicians may become detached in an attempt to avoid dealing with the difficult emotional aspects of death and dying. There is no predicting how a particular patient or family will deal with hearing bad news. The protective barrier of professional distance can become a wall that is impenetrable for those we care for. Only after dealing with personal feelings about death and dying can providers avoid nontherapeutic responses to patients with such a prognosis. The natural response to patients with difficult medical conditions is difficult enough, without adding unfinished business on the part of the provider, which most certainly will interfere with the ability to be therapeutic. Working with a partner or in pair formation in a simulated clinical scenario may be a valuable method of gaining confidence in this area as well as decreasing feelings of isolation for the clinician (Wakefield, Cooke, & Boggis, 2003). Special attention to providing a comfortable environment, taking enough time with the patient, and utilizing an empathetic approach is most effective (Ptacek & Ptacek, 2001).

Models

One model for communicating bad news has been described by Faulkner (1998). In this model, clinicians need to prepare beforehand in terms of planning both the provision of privacy and lack of interruptions. This includes thinking about the ideal setting for the delivery of the news. It is also important to think about who should be present beyond the immediate patient. Step 2 involves identifying what the patient knows or suspects. It is suggested that the clinician give an initial warning statement in order to communicate that the news is serious or difficult.

In step 3, attention is paid to the pace of providing information in order to make certain that the patient is not missing important news as a result of being overwhelmed. In order to be assured that the patient is clear about what is being said, the clinician needs to ask the patient to relay what they have heard being said about diagnosis, treatment, and prognosis. It is a mistake to continue to provide information if the patient cannot absorb it. Scheduling an additional appointment may be the best strategy when the patient has shut down and is unable to take in more information. Remember that the patient will not retain much after the initial news, so writing down information may be useful. During this stage the patient's reaction needs to be noted so that an appropriate intervention can be aimed at the individual patient. There are a variety of typical emotional reactions that can be expected including denial, blame, intellectualization, disbelief, and acceptance (Vandekieft, 2001). Identifying both verbal and nonverbal behavior is required in order to accurately assess the patient's response to the news. Validation is the communication strategy that is utilized to make certain your assessment is valid. Use of an empathetic response is appropriate, along with the mandate of providing realistic hope for the patient and family.

In step 4, the clinician assesses the patient's need for "space" before additional information is provided. Does the patient and family need time alone in order to absorb the news?

In step 5, the clinician identifies the patient's concerns and answers questions that the patient or family might have at this point. Taking a leadership role in guiding the interaction, the clinician needs to map a treatment plan for the patient. It is also the time to provide contact information and additional community resources for the patient and family.

Buckman (1992) has developed a six-step protocol for breaking bad news to patients. The steps include:

1. Getting started by assuring a private setting and allowing the patient to decide who should be present.
2. Finding out how much the patient knows. Inquire what the patient has already been told about the diagnosis and how much the patient understands about what has been told to them. Assess the patient's level of technical understanding as well as their emotional state.
3. Finding out how much the patient wants to know. Ask the patient what level of detail they desire, establishing there is no one right way for this conversation to follow.
4. Sharing the information. The clinician needs to have planned ahead of time and have the relevant information on hand. Topics to consider include diagnosis, course of treatment, prognosis, and resources for support. It is important to avoid using medical jargon and avoid lecturing the patient and family.
5. Responding to the patient's feelings. Identify and acknowledge the patient's emotional responses.
6. Planning and follow-through. Summarize the patient's concerns and medical issues. A careful and detail plan should include the next steps and plans for future contacts with the patient as well as information about referral providers and how the patient should proceed if questions arise in the future.

An abbreviated comparison of these two models can be seen in Table 6-1.

Table 6-1 Models for Communicating Bad News

Faulker (1998)	Buckman (1992)
Step 1: Plan for appropriate setting in which to delivery the news	Step 1: Private setting with appropriate people in attendance
Step 2: Identify patient's level of knowledge or understanding of the situation	Step 2: Find out how much patient knows
Step 3: Pace yourself to ensure patient/family understands	Step 3: Find out how much patient wants to know
Step 4: Assess patient's need for time to absorb the news	Step 4: Share the information
Step 5: Identify patient's concerns and answer questions	Step 5: Respond to patient's feelings/reaction
	Step 6: Develop a plan for future contact and referral information, if needed

Lessons from Oncology

Parker et al. (2001) found that patients find message content an important component of difficult conversations about their cancer diagnosis and management, although supportive and facilitative aspects of the discussion were equally valued. Understanding what is important to patients when told news about their cancer provides valuable information that may help refine how this challenging task is best performed.

Hagerty et al. (2004) found that metastatic cancer patients desire detailed information about symptoms, treatments, and side effects. In particular, they want information about "survival time." In a later study, Hagerty et al. (2005) found that patients wanted doctors to be realistic and to provide an opportunity to ask questions and treat them as individuals. The study found that the clinicians who were current in regard to treatment options and who offered hope in regard to pain control engendered a sense of hope. In contrast, those who seemed nervous and used euphemisms did the opposite. Realism and individualizing care were identified as key elements as well as a clinical style of being the expert, while emphasizing a positive attitude and being collaborative when dealing with the patient.

The cancer survivorship and agency model (O'Hair et al., 2003) has identified stages that can serve as a guide to the clinician in regard to tailoring communication according to the needs of patients and families. The stages are:

- Shock
- Uncertainty
- Empowerment
- Agency

Shock

The initial stage of shock is entered upon hearing the diagnosis of cancer, and consists of confusion and is often accompanied by fear. Not only do patients need to enter into a new world of medical terminology, but they must make choices about complicated treatments that will affect the rest of their lives. The proper psychological term for this stage is acute stress reaction, first described during the 1920s by Walter Cannon (Cannon, 1929). The initial theory was later developed as the first stage of a general adaptation syndrome related to stress response. During this response the sympathetic nervous system is involved, due to the involvement of the adrenal glands and the secretion of epinephrine and nonepinephrine. Physical symptoms include increased heart rate and respiration while the flight-or-fight response is triggered.

Acute stress disorder is a psychiatric diagnosis that is defined in the *Diagnostic and Statistical Manual of Mental Disorders (DSM IV)* as a set of symptoms following a traumatic event. These include: experiencing at least three dissociative symptoms; with at least one intrusion, avoidance or hyperarousal symptom. In addition, these symptoms must affect the patient's functioning and persist from 2 to 28 days (American Psychiatric Association, 1994). Nonpsychiatric clinicians need to be alert to patient reports of experiencing intrusive thoughts, flashbacks, withdrawal, or difficulty sleeping and startle response as they may relate to this diagnosis as effects of being informed of a diagnosis. The differential diagnosis between acute stress reaction and disorder will probably be made by a primary care provider, but can be easily missed if specific follow-up questions are not posed to the patient in subsequent visits.

The initial stage of shock is often within the context of having to wait for test results over days or weeks. The patient may have been experiencing vague symptoms, such as feeling tired or have pain in a certain part of their body, that have caused them to worry. Patients may vary in response to seeking clarification of a symptom, some dismissing it and others seeking help quickly. Regardless of how soon the patient sought care, the reality of having to wait for lab results, a mammogram, a biopsy, etc., can be excruciating. This is the backdrop of telling the patient the news of having a cancer diagnosis. Patients may not share with family members until the results of tests are revealed. Even though the patient and family might have worried about such a diagnosis, the news is met with shock.

The most important aspect of communication during this stage is to realize that the patient and family will not be able to process great amounts of information at this point. Information overload will occur if the clinician gets ahead of the patient and family. Acknowledgment of the felt experience of the news (feeling upset, confused, or even numb) is appropriate, and a focus on what needs to occur next is useful. Most of the time additional testing will be recommended as a next step, and sensitivity to scheduling this as soon as possible seems only humane.

To validate this emotional reaction can be normalizing for the patient, as they come to understand that typically patients have an initial reaction that will shift after a period of time.

Uncertainty

The concept of uncertainty is a major component in most types of illness. In an interesting analysis of the concept of uncertainty, Babrow, Kasch, and Ford (1998) identified various forms of uncertainty. These include: complexity; quality of information; probability; information structure; and beliefs about what can be known in general about life. Not only are many illnesses' trajectories uncertain due to the complexity of the illness, but the type of information that patients and families receive and how clear and complete that information is also affects issues of uncertainty. The beliefs of the patient and family in regard to

---

Box 6-1   Implications of Uncertainty for the Healthcare Provider

Assess the level of complexity of the illness
Assess the cognitive ability of the receiver
Assess the current understanding of the illness
Avoid using vague language or jargon
Focus on relevant information and avoid overloading the patient
Assess the amount of ambiguity inherent in the particular illness
Avoid communicating inconsistent or contradictory information
Understand the meaning of uncertainly to the patient and family

probability will combine with their beliefs and values as they struggle to integrate new information provided by healthcare professionals. How is the experience of a family member's diagnosis of a chronic or terminal illness to be understood and processed? How does the cold reality of a medical diagnosis and what course it will take fit with an overall understanding of how life operates in regard to certainty or uncertainty?

The implications for the healthcare provider regarding what we know about uncertainty are in Box 6-1.

Empowerment

The concept of empowerment began to be discussed first in the natural health-care arena. The explosion of the Internet, along with the demands for cost containment, have fueled the concept. It involves who makes decisions regarding health and treatment issues, whether the medical condition is chronic illness or pain management (Weiner, 2003). The goal of empowering patients and families is predicated on the need to provide information to the patient in regard to their illness or disease. It is also an aspect of patient-focused care, in that the patient's needs and concerns remain the center of care and communications. Patients are informed and then given choices in relation to their treatment and care. Patient education does not mean only providing knowledge in regard to a specific disease but rather, educating the patient in terms of decision-making (Santuri, 2006). Patients need to make decisions not only in terms of an illness, but also in terms of how the medical condition might affect their roles of parent, partner, employee, etc., as well as considering the psychologic impact of the illness.

The concept of empowerment is in tune with a wider political and cultural emphasis on individual choice, and gains validity from psychological research and theory that attests to the superiority of ways of coping with challenges—including illness or treatment—that exert control over the challenge (Guadagnoli, 1998). Studies of cancer patients reveal that they value being given information as a way of building relationships with clinicians and as a way of maintaining hope (Salander, 2002).

Critics of patient empowerment warn that, carried too far, the model excuses healthcare providers from their responsibility (Salmon, Phil, & Hall, 2004). While evidence-based research on empowerment is still in its infancy, the spirit of the concept aligns with the patient-centered approach to health care.

Healthcare and disease information is no longer only available to those in the healthcare professions. The patient as consumer is now able to access dozens of Web sites that address their health concern. Search engines make information available at no cost from the privacy of the patient's home. But with access and availability comes a need for evaluating the quality and accuracy of the information. Patients will have varying educational levels and language skills. It is not always clear what Web sites offer information versus advertising for certain products. What is the role of the clinician in the midst of this information glut? The provider as gatekeeper and guide seem to be roles that the advanced practice nurse is well suited to assume. As a result of an assessment of the learning needs and abilities of patients and families, the clinician is in a good position to suggest valid informational resources. While brochures may be available for dissemination to patients, the provider needs to consider the source and evaluate them for accuracy of content and appropriateness for a particular patient or family. Web sites, developed by patients, may be useful and accurate, or bias and disturbing if graphic discussions are held regarding one particular treatment versus another. Only by knowing the particular patient or family can the clinician recommend which Web sites might be helpful, and it means that the provider will need to stay abreast of what is offered on the Web to both recommend to view and recommend to avoid. Patients will most certainly need and want information in regard to various therapies, and once again, the relationship with the provider can be a powerful foundation to receiving and evaluating this information.

Agency

This term refers to the process of patients understanding choices and feeling competent to act on the choices. Working with a patient in this stage involves responding to their concerns and questions and respecting their decisions. This may mean dealing with issues of pain management, hospice care, chemotherapy, or palliative care. Patients may feel more comfortable expressing such issues if their experience up to that point has been supportive and respectful. It requires that the clinician identify to the patient a bias, if one exists, for one alternative over another and provide the supporting data that underlies a preference. It also requires acknowledgment that, ultimately, it is the patient's choice that is paramount, even if it disagrees with your opinion or the wishes of family members.

The care of the terminally ill patient needs to not only take into account the various barriers to good communication in this situation, but also focus on a plan of care that centers on the needs of the patient. Lo, Quill, and Tulsky (1999) offer a guide for initiating conversations about end-of-life care. They suggest inquiring about:

- What the concerns are for the patient and family
- How the patient and family feel the treatment is going
- What the patient and family view as the worst thing that could happen
- What the best thing that could happen might be
- What has been most difficult about the illness to date
- What the patient's and family's hopes are
- What the most important when thinking about the future is

The topic of a patient and family's relationship to spirituality is also important to assess. Regardless of the spiritual affiliation or belief system of the provider, specific questions need to be initiated by the clinician without judgment or bias. Asking patients and families if they have a spiritual framework that guides or assists them is a neutral way to open up this conversation. If the answer is "no," then the clinician need not go any further. If the patient does have a framework, the clinician can inquire about how their belief system has assisted them in the past and if there are individuals who could be called on for assistance at this time. A patient's beliefs about life-after-death may be consoling, as they may believe they will reunite with loved ones who have died. Acknowledging that life is coming to an end may prompt a discussion about any unfinished business the patient may have. This may be in the form of conducting conversations with friends or family members or accomplishing realistic goals that may be unmet. Travel plans may be instituted, if the patient is able, to fulfill life dreams, for example. Final visits to family that may live some distance away from the patient might need to be arranged.

When reviewing their life, patients may express regret about certain aspects of their life. They may feel they were not a good parent or adequate son or daughter. A patient may express regret that they were not faithful in a relationship or honest in their business dealings. The role of the clinician in this situation is to *listen* and allow the patient to have regrets. While reassuring patients that they did their best may make the clinician feel supportive and a bit better, it is far more therapeutic to allow the patient to express what they may regret at the end of life. Life review is a common process and it will not be uncommon for any of us to have some regret at life's end. This is another example of reassurance not being the best response by the provider. Validation about what the patient is saying in a neutral manner is far more healing. In that way, the clinician serves as witness and will not fall into the trap of being dismissive by brushing away the patient's real and valid feelings.

Hope

Fully informing patients and families about limited life expectancy and maintaining a positive attitude and a sense of hope would seem to be a balancing act. Both clinicians and patients express the need for maintaining hope (Nowotny, 1991; Sardell & Trierweiler, 1993). Truth-telling has been studied in this context and findings suggest that clinicians report a fear of robbing patients of hope if they are told the truth (Glass & Douglas, 2004). In order to sustain truth-telling, an important issue for the nurse–patient relationship, qualities of honesty, justice, and courage will be required (Hodkinson, 2008). In one study, the themes of controlling symptoms—receiving emotional support, care, and dignity; identifying realistic goals; and discussions about day-to-day living—were identified as helping patients maintain hope and strengthen coping skills (Clayton, Butow, Arnold, & Tattersall, 2005). Historically, nurses have been reluctant to tell patients the truth about their medical condition and have been accused of favoring a communication style that values control of the clinical encounter as opposed to attending to the best interests of the patient (Tuckett, 2005). The notion that terminally ill patients will lose hope if they are told the specifics of their situation is refuted by the evidence (Brooksbank & Cassell, 2005). While patients may lose hope that is related to recovery or cure, they need to retain the hope of accomplishing whatever is reasonable and important for the time that they have left. Relationships may need to be repaired, patients may need to connect with important friends and family members in order to give final goodbyes, and patients may need to come to grips with a particular spiritual framework in order to make final preparations for death. Patients may need to borrow the hope of accomplishing these tasks from clinicians who are caring for them while they attempt to reach a level of acceptance of their clinical reality. Caregivers can also encourage patients to initiate conversations with loved ones that will either heal or say goodbye.

Talking to patients who have cancer or other terminal diseases is not the only category of difficult clinical conversations. While students may avoid these conversations in their clinical rotations, they are bound to arise in everyday practice. Discussing sexual matters may be challenging for both the patient and the provider.

Communications Following Miscarriage

Emotional reactions following miscarriage fall into the general category of grief reactions (Brier, 2008) and, therefore, communication strategies are similar to those utilized when working with patients coping with significant loss. Clinicians need to assist patients in identifying and verbalizing the *meaning* of the loss, both real and symbolic, and then develop a plan based on this meaning. The psychologic sequelae of miscarriage also include guilt, loss of a part of self, and a change in personal identity (Frost & Condon, 1996). These issues may also have serious implications for a patient's family members who may require intervention, as miscarriage is a family event.

Communication About Sexual Functioning

Not all difficult conversations are as a result of a serious diagnosis of cancer or a terminal illness. The area of sexual functioning may pose unease in the patient, the provider, or both. Surveys in general medical practice report that between 10 and 15% of patients experience a sexual problem (Myerscough, Ford, Myerscough, & Currie, 1996). Sexual conversations may occur in a variety of situations. They may be a part of a routine history or arise as a result of discussing the side effects of a medication. They may be the primary reason for the office visit, such as seeking contraception or concerns about decreased libido or problems with vaginal dryness during menopause and thereafter. Whether a patient will openly discuss their questions and concerns depends in part on their comfort with their sexuality, the relationship with the provider, and the perceived comfort the patient assesses in the provider in discussing these matters. If a patient is worried about having contracted a sexually transmitted disease, they may also worry about the judgment of the provider. If a patient makes a visit to receive a pregnancy test the clinician may not know the circumstances that surround the possible pregnancy. The patient may present with a chronic disease, such as multiple sclerosis, in which sexual activity is affected. A patient may secretly be worried about an inability to orgasm and hope that the clinician asks about sexual functioning and have information and suggestions. A patient experiencing marital problems, which are translated into a lack of sexual activity, may need to discuss the issue and get a referral for couples therapy. An adolescent has decided to begin a sexual relationship with her boyfriend, but requests birth control to treat acne. A patient who has experienced recent bowel surgery and resultant stoma is concerned about how his sexual life will be managed.

The first step the clinician needs to take is to be clear about their personal beliefs about sexual issues. What is your position in regard to the timing of adolescent sexual behavior? What attitudes do you have concerning abortion? Does this position differ if the woman is a teen, married, or is a victim of sexual abuse or rape? What are your beliefs about sexual activity as one ages? The reason that the provider must be clear about their beliefs is that unrecognized beliefs may taint the relationship with the patient and interfere with a therapeutic aspect of the relationship. One of the challenges of maintaining a therapeutic relationship is the ability to put aside one's personal views and keep the patient and their belief system and their concerns as the focus. Patients and families will not always make choices that jive with the clinician's views. By recognizing our personal beliefs, we can more easily set them aside and attend to the patient.

Considering the myriad of ways that sexual conversations can occur, it is advised to develop a comfort level with initiating sexual communications in case patients are too anxious or hesitant to do so. Sexual functioning certainly should be noted in a complete physical exam, and sexual activity discussed in subsequent annual visits. Being direct and conveying an ease with the topic is the strategy, after an initial rapport with the patient is established. If the patient has identified a sexual problem then the inquiry follows according to the complaint. If, on the other hand, the provider has questions about sexual functioning based on other issues that the patient has discussed, the inquiry should be done with a neutral and matter-of-fact inquiry. It is most important to never make assumptions in regard to sexual activity of a patient at any age and regardless of marital status or sexual identity. Asking, as opposed to assuming, is the general rule. Becoming comfortable with discussing sexual topics is a matter of practice. It is my experience that graduate nursing students have little experience with this area, beyond the brief mention of sexual functioning accomplished in the physical examination. Learning how to phrase a clinical inquiry in your own words is the solution to the discomfort experienced by most novices.

Patients will sometimes wait for the provider to open up this line of inquiry. If the provider can convey a level of comfort with this subject that is free from judgment, the patient may be able to share private concerns about sexual functioning. The provider also needs to be familiar with resources that may assist a patient with their concerns. Good information is available in regard to sexual dysfunction including premature ejaculation, impotence, sexual unresponsiveness, and vaginismus. Providers need to be familiar with the literature as well as clinicians in the area who treat sexual dysfunction.

Talking to patients about sexually transmitted diseases may be the primary reason for a patient visit or occur during a visit that has an entirely different focus. Because of the sensitivity of the topic, patients may be particularly worried about being judged or issues of confidentiality. In the era of AIDS some patients may wish to be tested, but hold back due to fear of finding out the facts. At times the provider will need to take the lead and suggest testing and be available when the results are determined. Again, community resources for support will provide invaluable information and support for patients and families.

Communication About Alcohol and Substance Abuse

In recent years the abuse of drugs and alcohol has been studied under the umbrella of risky health behaviors. When considering preventive health care, the abuse of alcohol and drugs is listed along with cigarette smoking and obesity. Primary care would seem to be the natural setting for identifying patients who are jeopardizing their health by engaging in these behaviors and the setting to begin to address changing these risky behaviors. Primary care clinicians are often the first point of contact within the healthcare system for patients. While issues related to risky health behavior may not be the identified reason for a clinical visit, these clinical encounters present an opportunity in regard to both preventative care and treatment. Both patients and clinicians may find it difficult to discuss alcohol or drug abuse, even when it is suspected. However, many common patient complaints seen in primary care, including diabetes, sleep disorders, anxiety, gastrointestinal disturbances, depression, hypertension, and asthma, may be alcohol related. If nothing else, a combination of these disorders with alcohol or drug use makes clinical management more difficult. Routine screening for risky health behaviors opens channels of communication between patients and providers and sets the stage for interventions or referrals.

Although there are a variety of screening tools for both use of alcohol and drugs, the actual rates of screening are troubling. In one study, while the majority of patients reported having a risk factor (typically overweight), only 29% reported being screened and, of those who were screened, issues of physical activity and smoking were identified, over diet and use of alcohol (Coups, Gaba, & Orleans, 2004). Current thinking in both preventive care and primary care circles is a need for the development of a screening tool to address *multiple* risk factors during the primary care visit, while acknowledging the time crunch that exists during a typical clinical visit. Reconfiguring the typical primary care visit would mean a collaboration of various stakeholders, including patients, clinicians, payors, and healthcare policy leaders (Babor, Sciamanna, & Pronk, 2004). A criticism of current screening tools is the fact that they only focus on one risky health behavior. The Prescription for Health, a Robert Wood Johnson Foundation program in conjunction with the Agency for Healthcare Research and Quality, conducted a study of a large number of practice networks in an effort to test a tool that would address four risky health behaviors and assess efficacy of health behavior change (Glasgow et al., 2005). The risky behaviors being assessed included lack of physical activity, risky drinking, smoking, and eating patterns. Recommended assessment tools for each of the identified four health risk behaviors can be found online at http://www.annfammed.org.

Babor et al. (2004) identify a variety of available screening tools including the Drug Abuse Screening Test (DAST), the CAGE-AID, the Substance Abuse Screening Instrument (SASI), and the World Health Organization Alcohol, Smoking, and Substance Involvement Screening Test (ASSIST). These are self-reporting tests and have the problem of not having severity measurements, are not specific, and do not differentiate between lifetime and current use. For adolescents there are the Problem-Oriented Screening Instrument for Teenagers (POSIT), the Drug Use Screening Inventory (DUSI), the Personal Experience Screening Questionnaire (PESQ), and the Drug and Alcohol Problem (DAP) Quick Screen. These are lengthy and not easy to administer. Other tests include the MacAndrew Alcoholism Scale (MAC), the Addiction Potential Scale (APS), and the Substance Abuse Subtle Screening Inventory (SASSI). These scales identify factors that might lead an individual to go on to drug abuse but are not highly sensitive or specific and, therefore, not generally recommended for use in primary care.

Beyond self-report surveys and indirect self-reports are typical tests including hair testing, urinalysis, and blood and saliva testing. While easy to perform, they are prone to be subject to false-negatives and introduce conflict and tension into the provider–patient relationship. In addition to consequences for the therapeutic relationship, there are legal and ethical constraints. Babor et al. (2004) raise the question of whether drug screening might be best accomplished by a "Trojan horse" approach, which would integrate drug screening with alcohol, tobacco, diet, and exercise screening. This strategy would seem to me to have major ramifications for the therapeutic relationship, as well as legal and ethical concerns. Babor does make the point that the choice of a screening tool are less important than the process of doing a screening, which relays the importance of the ongoing monitoring of risky health behaviors to a patient. Steinweg and Worth (1993) found that using open-ended questions when administering the CAGE screening tool "dramatically enhanced" its sensitivity. In addition, sensitivity was severely reduced when providers focused on the quantitative data relating to amount and frequency of alcohol use.

When developing a strategy regarding *how* to talk to a patient about addiction, Karno and Longabaugh (2005) found that with patients who are resistant to the idea of changing drinking behavior the clinician should avoid giving information or advice. Instead, encouraging patients to talk about what is most important to them, and *listening* is the best approach.

Addictions are chronic conditions in which relapse is more common and expected than not. In primary care settings the clinician needs to develop an acceptance of this reality, in order to avoid countertransference responses to patients who relapse. In addition developing a strategy to prevent relapse, Friedmann, Saitz, and Samet (1998) have identified the following elements:

- Supportive therapeutic relationship
- Scheduling regular follow-up visits
- Getting the patient's extended family involved
- Recommending active involvement in a 12-step program
- Assist the patient in developing a plan to manage relapses
- Assist the patient in identifying triggers
- Assist the patient in developing coping strategies
- Management of comorbid conditions (depression, anxiety)
- Consider psychopharmacology intervention
- Collaborate with addiction providers

Stages of Change

When considering the best approach to utilize when talking to patients about addictive behavior, it is useful to remember stages of change as outlined by Prochaska et al. (1994). Assessment of the stages of change, on a continuum, shows the patient will determine how the topic is discussed. Like any continuum, patients move back and forth among the various stages depending on a variety of factors related to the cost/benefit of behaviors. It is during the stage of contemplation, characterized by ambivalence, that change occurs most often. If the provider uses a confrontational approach when the patient is in the stage of precontemplation, then resistance to the idea of change will most probably result. The goals of any clinical visit need to be moving the patient along the continuum of change (Burge & Schneider, 1999). The process of assessment can be the beginning point of self-reflection in regard to use of alcohol or drugs. It is only with patients who require immediate change, such as pregnant patients, who require a firm direct approach. Even in this situation, providing information about alcoholism or community resources rather than advice is preferred. A nondirective approach decreases the chance of resistance on the part of the patient as they weigh the personal costs and benefits of alcohol use in their life.

Communication and Behavioral Change

Frequently, healthcare providers will find themselves in a position of encouraging health promotion and illness prevention when talking to patients and families. Behaviors associated with these areas of concern are usually behaviors related to lifestyle. In *Healthy People 2010*, the leading health indicators include physical activity, obesity, smoking, drug abuse, sexual behavior, mental health, violence, injury, quality of the environment, and access to health care (US Department of Health & Human Services, 2000). One of the identified goals is to "use communication strategically to improve health." Subsumed under this goal are issues related to health literacy, use of the Internet for health information, creation of centers of excellence, and patient satisfaction with healthcare provider's communication skills.

Van Servellen (2009) summarizes the principles of change theory that relate to changing health behavior. These include:

- Change is incremental and dynamic by its nature.
- Motivation to change must be internalized in order for the change to be permanent.

- Reinforcement of behavior is motivating and can be either positive or negative.
- Motivation to change is linked to a perceived need to change on the part of the patient.
- Social support systems have a direct effect on desire to change and in sustaining behavioral change.
- Patients must believe in their ability to change behavior.
- Support and confidence in the patient enhance behavioral change.

These principles highlight the communication skills required for the clinician in regard to patient interactions. These include the ability to provide support, positive reinforcement, encouragement, and overall belief in the patient in their attempt to make lifestyle changes. They also underscore the requirement that the provider be nonjudgmental and exhibit patience. The road to making health behavior changes is inherently difficult. As healthcare providers we all know how much sleep we ought to get each night, how we ought to exercise regularly, and how we ought to eat. Knowing these facts is simply not enough. It is the implementation that is difficult, and lifestyle changes are challenging. By realizing how complex and challenging this process is, providers will be able to be empathic and gentle when patients struggle or fail. It may take time to fully incorporate a need for change or to believe it is possible. The support of one's healthcare provider will facilitate the process of change.

COMMUNICATION EXERCISES

1. Difficult Conversations

Pair off as patient and provider.

The clinical scenario is that the patient has had a lung x-ray that detected a spot on his/her lung. You are meeting to discuss these findings and plan the next course of action.

Provider:

Proceed with the meeting with a style of denial, giving the patient little information and being vague and using medical terms. Focus only on the physical aspects of the situation, ignoring the emotional response the patient has.

Do a second interview, being clear and tuning into the patient's emotional as well as physical concerns.

Discussion:

Share your perspectives, as both provider and patient.

How were the two interviews different?

What issues arose for the provider? For the patient?

Share with one another situations that you have participated in that are similar to this situation.

What might you do differently in future clinical encounters?

_____

_____

_____

_____

_____

_____

_____

_____

2. Difficult Conversations

Pair off as patient and provider.

Provider:

You are meeting with a long-standing patient to discuss the metastasis of a formerly treated breast cancer.

Patient:

Introduce into the dialogue a lack of hope and fear of dying.

Discussion:

Share what each role was like.

Share how comfortable your provider seemed to be with the issue of death and how they responded to your loss of hope.

As the provider, examine your comfort level with the topic.

What strategies did you think were particularly effective?

What was ineffective?

What would you do differently in future?

What feelings do you have about this type of clinical encounter?

_____

_____

_____

_____

_____

_____

_____

_____

3. Sexual History

Group as patient, provider, and observer.

Provider:

Conduct the portion of the interview that deals with sexual history.

Patient:

You are a divorced 34-year-old woman who has recently begun dating after a difficult divorce.

Observer:

Note body language of the provider as she/he conducts the interview.

Record open and closed questions.

Document questions that caused the patient to open up to the provider.

Discussion:

Observer, share your observations with patient and provider.

Provider, share your experience in conducting this interview.

Patient, share what aspects of the interview you felt were effective and ineffective.

Switch roles.

_____

_____

_____

_____

_____

_____

_____

_____

4. Obesity

Pair off as patient and provider: 30 minutes.

Provider:

This is your first appointment with a 45-year-old woman, who you are see-ing for a routine physical examination for work. You steer the interview to the issue of the patient's weight. Be aware of your use of both open and closed questions.

Patient:

You are a 45-year-old woman, whose weight is 257 lbs. You have strug-gled with your weight for your entire life, and have been unsuccessful in maintaining a normal weight. You have tried many fad diets, and even re-sorted to not eating at times in your life. You feel ashamed of yourself and hopeless about this situation.

Discussion:

Share your perspectives on the interview.

What were the difficulties during the interview?

What components of the interview were effective?

What would have improved the interview?

What personal emotions get stirred up when dealing with this topic?

_____

_____

_____

_____

_____

_____

_____

5. Alcohol Abuse

Pair off as patient and provider: 30 minutes.

Provider:

Proceed with a clinical encounter related to a routine annual clinical visit.

Patient:

You are concerned about your consumption of alcohol, which has increased due to current stressors of losing your job. You hope to discuss this with your provider at your next annual physical visit.

Discussion:

After 20 minutes, share how the encounter unfolded and how successful it was in relation to the patient sharing with the provider his/her concern about alcohol.

What could have been improved?

What was most effective?

What can you use of this experience in your next clinical encounters?

_____

_____

_____

_____

_____

_____

_____

_____

6. Drug Abuse

Pair off as patient and provider: 30 minutes.

Provider:

You see that the chief complaint for this patient is back pain, and note on the chart that he/she has a history of drug abuse.

Patient:

You recently were involved in a car accident and have been experiencing severe back pain.

Discussion:

Share your two perspectives as provider and patient with one another.

What biases or concerns played a part in the interaction?

What were the stumbling blocks, if any?

Assess how satisfying the interactions was from both the perspective of the patient and the provider.

How could this interaction have been improved?

What are the lessons you can take into the clinical setting with patients?

_____

_____

_____

_____

_____

_____

_____

_____

JOURNALING EXERCISES

1. Difficult Conversations

Describe the most difficult clinical conversation you have had to date.

What made it most challenging?

Describe your assessment of your skills at the time of the interaction.

What part of the interaction went better than expected, if any?

How would you approach a similar situation today?

What about your approach is different than the past encounter?

Share this with a colleague.

_____

_____

_____

_____

_____

_____

_____

_____

2. Shock

Recall a clinical encounter where the patient or family had an acute stress reaction.

Describe how you felt during the interaction.

What was your response to the patient or family?

Would you handle the situation differently today?

Describe what thoughts you have about this clinical encounter.

How does this interaction inform you and represent learning for future similar situations?

_____

_____

_____

_____

_____

_____

_____

_____

3. Sexual Issues

Describe your current beliefs and understanding about sexual identity.

How did you happen to develop these views?

Are there difficult patient encounters that have taxed your belief system?

If so, describe them and why they were difficult.

Which issues in this area do you still struggle with?

What do you believe can best guide an advanced practice clinician in regard to these issues?

_____

_____

_____

_____

_____

_____

_____

4. Patients With Terminal Illness

Have you ever been in the position of delivering bad news in this area?

Have you been present when someone else delivered the news?

Describe either or both of the previous, identifying what your internal reaction was at the time and after.

What part of the conversation was most difficult?

What changes would you make in future when engaging in similar conversations?

Was there an opportunity to interact with the patient's family?

If so, describe this interaction and how it differed from the conversation with the patient.

What resources were and are currently available to you in regard to caring for yourself in these situations?

_____
_____
_____
_____
_____
_____
_____
_____

5. Sexual Functioning

What do you think is an appropriate age for the beginning of sexual activity?

What do you think is the appropriate age for the cessation of sexual activity?

How have these beliefs played out in your life?

If you have children, particularly adolescents, what has been the challenge in this area as a parent?

If you have aging parents, has the issue of sexual activity come up?

Describe your current situation in regard to sexual functioning.

How might your current situation present challenges or advantages in your professional life?

Describe any examples of either of the previous scenarios.

_____
_____
_____
_____
_____
_____
_____
_____

6. Patient Adherence/Compliance

Define the concepts of adherence and compliance.

Do you think there is a difference in these words?

Describe several experiences of working with patients who have been labeled as noncompliant.

What behavior on the part of staff did you observe when working with or discussing a noncompliant patient?

What ideas do you have regarding dealing with this patient?

How will you transfer this awareness when working with patients in the future?

_____

_____

_____

_____

_____

_____

_____

_____

7. Patient Compliance/Adherence

Discuss any experience you have with patients who have chosen to not adhere to a treatment plan or medication regime recommended by your preceptor or yourself.

Describe any internal "buttons" that were pushed for you.

How do you respond to patients who do not follow treatment recommendations in general?

What conversations have you had with patients regarding nonadherence?

What challenges do these patients present for you?

What ideas do you have when working with this population?

_____

_____

_____

_____

_____

_____

_____

_____

8. Compliance/Adherence

Describe your philosophy of who is responsible for a patient's health.

How did you develop this stance?

What challenges does this philosophy present for you?

How has this position changed over time, if it has?

Are there ethical issues related to your philosophy?

What are the legal implications of your philosophy?

Do you feel that health care is a right or a privilege?

Defend this position.

What are the implications of this position as an advanced practice nurse?

What are the challenges?

_____

_____

_____

_____

_____

_____

_____

9. Alcohol/Drug Abuse

Identify an individual in your family or origin who has a problem with alcohol or drugs.

Identify any individual in your immediate circle, current spouse or partner and friends, who have a problem with alcohol.

How has interacting with these people affected you in general?

How have these relationships affected your view of people who abuse alcohol or drugs?

Explain how these relationships affect your personal life.

What are the areas of vulnerability and strength that have evolved out of this history?

Document a clinical encounter with a patient who is in recovery or an active alcoholic.

What were the challenges of this interaction?

Identify your thoughts regarding your effectiveness.

Identify your feelings about this clinical encounter.

What was your strategy in regard to stages of change theory?

_____

_____

_____

_____

_____

_____

_____

_____

10. Changing Health Behavior

How would you assess your health according to the objectives of *Healthy People 2010*?

What have been the challenges you have faced in regard to any of your personal issues?

What role has your primary care provider played in assisting you in these goals?

Describe your readiness to change in regard to Prochaska's stages.

Discuss what would be useful for you in order to reach your goals.

How could you apply this learning to your professional encounters with patients?

_____

_____

_____

_____

_____

_____

_____

_____

11. Working with Addiction

Document your experience of working with patients who have been labeled as drug seeking.

What are your thoughts about these patients?

What are your feelings about these patients?

Describe the reactions you have observed from peers when work with patients with a history of addiction.

What strategy do you employ when working with this population?

Identify the effectiveness of the strategy.

_____

_____

_____

_____

_____

_____

_____

REFERENCES

American Psychiatric Association. *Diagnostic and statistical manual of mental disorders* (4th ed.). (1994). Washington, DC: Author.

Babrow, A., Kasch, C., & Ford, L. (1998). The many meanings of "uncertainty" in illness. *Health Communications, 10,* 1–24.

Baile, W. (2000). *Report of the NCCN Task Force on Physician-Patient Communication.* Paper presented at the annual conference of the National Comprehensive Cancer Network, Fort Lauderdale, FL.

Babor, T. F., Sciamanna, C. N., & Pronk, N. P. (2004). Assessing multiple risk behaviors in primary care. *American Journal of Preventitive Medicine, 27*(2S), 42–53.

Barnard, D. (1995). The promise of intimacy and the fear of our own undoing. *Journal of Palliative Care, 11*(4), 22–26.

Brooksbank, M. A., & Cassell, E. J. (2005). The place of hope in clinical medicine. In J. A. Elliott (Ed.), *Interdisciplinary perspectives on hope* (pp. 231–239). Hauppauge, New York: Nova Sciences.

Browning, D. (2003). To show our humanness. *Bioethics Forum, 18*(3–4), 23–28.

Brier, N. (2008). Grief following miscarriage: a comprehensive review of the literature. *Journal of Womens Health*, (Larchmont) *17*(3), 451–464.

Bruera, E., Palmer, J. L., Pace, E., Zhang, K., Wiley, J., Strasser, F., & Bennett, M. I. (2007). A randomized, controlled trial of physician postures when breaking bad news to cancer patients. *Palliative Medicine, 21*(6), 501–505.

Buckman, R. (1992). *How to break bad news*. Baltimore: John Hopkins University Press.

Burge, S. K., & Schneider, F. D. (1999). Alcohol-related problems: Recognition and intervention. *American Family Physician, 59*(2), 361–370, 372.

Butow, P. N., Dowsett, S., Hagerty, R. G., & Tattersall, M. H. (2002). Communicating prognosis to patients with metastatic disease: What do they really want to know? *Support Care Cancer, 10*, 161–168.

Cannon, W. (1929). *Bodily changes in pain, hunger, fear, and rage*. New York: Appleton.

Clayton, J. M., Butow, P. N., Arnold, R. M., & Tattersall, M. H. (2005). Fostering coping and nurturing hope when discussing the future with terminally ill cancer patients and their caregivers. *Cancer, 103*(9), 1965–1975.

Coulehan, J., & Block, M. (2001). *The medical interview*. Philadelphia: F. A. Davis.

Coups, E. J., Gaba, A., & Orleans, C. T. (2004). Physician screening for multiple behavioral health risk factors. *American Journal of Preventive Medicine, 27*(2S), 34–41.

de Haes, H., & Koedoot, N. (2003). Patient centered decision making in palliative cancer treatment: A world of paradoxes. *Patient and Educational Counseling, 50*(1), 43–49.

Derdiarian, A. K. (1986). Informational needs of recently diagnosed cancer patients. *Nursing Research, 35*, 276–281.

Faulkner, A. (1998). *When the news is bad*. Cheltenham, England: Stanley Thornes Ltd.

Fellowes, D., Wilkinson, S., & Moore, P. (2003). Communication skills training for health care professionals working with cancer patients, their families and/or carers. *Cochrane Database Systematic Review*, (2), CD003751.

Friedmann, P. D., Saitz, R., & Samet, J. H. (1998). Management of adults recovering from alcohol or other drug problems. *Journal of American Medical Association, 279*(15), 1227–1231.

Frost, M., & Condon, J. T. (1996). The psychological sequelae of miscarriage: A critical review of the literature. *Australia New Zealand Journal of Psychiatry, 30*(1), 54–62.

Glasgow, R. E., Ory, M. G., Klesges, L. M., Cifuentes, M., Fernald, D. H., & Green, L. A. (2005). Practical and relevant self-report measures of patient health behaviors for primary care research. *Annals of Family Medicine, 3*, 73–81.

Guadagnoli, E., & Ward, P. W. P. (1998). Patient participation in decision-making. *Social Science and Medicine, 47*, 329–339.

Glass, E., & Douglas, C. (2004). Truth-telling: Ethical issues in clinical practice. *Journal of Hospice and Palliative Nursing, 6*(4), 232–242.

Greisinger, A. J., Lorimor, R. J., Aday, L. A., Winn, R. J., & Baile, W. F. (1997). Terminally ill cancer patients: Their most important concerns. *Cancer Practice, 5*,147–154.

Hagerty, R. G., Butow, P. N., Ellis, P. A., Lobb, E. A., Pendlebury, S., Leighl, N., et al. (2004). Cancer patient preferences for communication of prognosis in the metastatic setting. *Journal of Clinical Oncology, 22*(9), 1721–1730.

Hagerty, R. G., Butow, P. N., Ellis, P. M., Lobb, E. A., Pendlebury, S. C., Leighl, N., et al. (2005). Communicating with realism and hope: Incurable cancer patients' views on the disclosure of prognosis. *Journal of Clinical Oncology, 23*(6), 1278–1288.

Hodkinson, K. (2008). How should a nurse approach truth-telling? A virtue ethics perspective. *Nursing Philosophy, 9*(4), 248–256.

Jenkins, V., Fallowfield, L., & Saul, J. (2001). Information needs of patients with cancer. *British Journal of Cancer, 81*(1), 48–51.

Karno, M. P., & Longabaugh, R. (2005). Less directiveness by therapists improves drinking outcomes of reactant clients in alcoholism treatment. *Journal of Consulting and Clinical Psychology, 73*(2), 262–267.

Kennedy Sheldon L. (2005). Communication in oncology care. *Clinical Journal of Oncology Nursing, 9*(3), 287.

Leydon, G. M., Boulton, M., Moynihan, C., Jones, A., Mossman, J., Boudioni, M., et al. (2000). Cancer patients' information needs and information seeking behaviour: In depth interview study. *British Medical Journal, 320*, 909–912.

Myerscough, P., & Ford, M. (1996). *Talking with patients: Keys to good communication.* New York: Oxford University Press.

Neuland, S. B. (1993). *How we die: Reflections on life's final chapter.* New York: Alfred A. Knopf.

Nowotny, M. L. (1991). Every tomorrow, a vision of hope. *Journal of Psychosocial Oncology, 9*(3), 117–126.

O'Hair, D., Villagran, M. M., Wittenberg, E., Brown, K., Ferguson, M., Hall, H. T. et al. (2003). Cancer survivorship and agency model. *Health Communications, 15*(2), 195–202.

Online Textbook. Retrieved May 26, 2009, from http://www.case.edu/med/epidbio/mphp439/Patient_Empowerment.htm

Parker, P. A., Baile, W. F., de Moor, C., Lenzi, R., Kudelka, A. P., & Cohen, L. (2001). Breaking bad news about cancer: Patients' preferences for communication. *Clinical Oncology, 19*, 2049–2056.

Pollak, K. I., Arnold, R. M., Jeffreys, A. S., Alexander, S.C., Olsen, M. K., Abernethy, A. P., et al. (2007). Oncologist communication about emotion during visits with patients with advanced cancer. *Journal of Clinical Oncology, 25*(36), 5748–5752.

Prochaska, J. O., Velicer, W. F., Rossi, J. S., Goldstein, M. G., Marcus, B. H., Rakowski, W., et al. (1994). Stages of change and decisional balance for 12 problem behaviors. *Health Psychology, 13*, 39–46.

Ptacek, J. T., & Ptacek, J. J. (2001). Patients' perceptions of receiving bad news about cancer. *Journal of Clinical Oncology, 19*, 4160–4164.

Lo, B., Quill, T., & Tulsky, J. (1999). Discussing palliative care with patients. *Annals of Internal Medicine, 130*, 744–749.

Razavi, D., & Delvaux, N. (1997). Communication skills and psychological training in oncology. *European Journal of Cancer, 33*(Suppl 6), S15–21.

Rosenzweig, M., Clifton, M., & Arnold, R. (2007). Development of communication skills workshop for oncology advanced practice nursing students. *Journal of Cancer Education, 22*(3), 149–153.

Salander, P. (2002). Bad news from the patient's perspective: An analysis of the written narratives of newly diagnosed cancer patients. *Social Science and Medicine, 55,* 721–732.

Salmon, P., & Hall, G. (2004). Patient empowerment or the emperor's new clothes. *Journal of Research and Social Medicine, 97*(2), 53–56.

Santuri, L. (2006). *Patient empowerment: Improving the outcomes of chronic diseases through self-management education.* Cleveland, OH: Case Western Reserve University.

Sardell, A., & Trierweiller, S. (1993) Disclosing the cancer diagnosis. *Cancer, 72,* 3355–3365.

Sapir, R., Catane, R., Kaufman, B., Isacson, R., Segal, A., Wein, S., et al. (2000). Cancer patient expectations of and communication with oncologists and oncology nurses: The experience of an integrated oncology and palliative care service. *Support Care Cancer, 8,* 458–463.

Sivesind, D., Parker, P. A., Cohen, L., Demoor, C., Bumbaugh, M., Throckmorton, T., et al. (2003). Communicating with patients in cancer care: What areas do nurses find most challenging? *Journal of Cancer Education, 18*(4), 202–209.

Steinweg, D. L., & Worth, H. (1993). Alcoholism: The keys to the CAGE. *American Journal of Medicine, 94*(5), 520–523.

Tuckett, A. G. (2005). The care encounter: Pondering caring, honest communication and control. *International Journal of Nursing Practice, 11*(2), 77–84.

US Department of Health and Human Services. *Tracking healthy people 2010.* (2000). Washington, DC: US Government Printing Office.

Van Servellen, G. (2009). Communication skills for the health professional. Sudbury, MA: Jones and Bartlett.

VandeKieft, G. K. (2001). Breaking bad news. *American Family Physician, 64*(12), 1975–1978.

Weiner, K. A. (2003). Empowering the pain patient to make treatment decisions. *Home Health Care Management and Practice, 15,* 198–202.

Wakefield, A., Cooke, S., & Boggis, C. (2003). Learning together: Use of simulated patients with nursing and medical students for breaking bad news. *International Journal of Palliative Nursing, 9*(1), 32–38.

SUGGESTED READINGS

Arnold, S., & Koczwara, B. (2006). Breaking bad news: Learning through experience. *Journal of Clinical Oncology, 24*(31), 5098–5100.

Beale, E., Baile, W., & Aaron, J. (2005). Silence is not golden: Communicating with children dying from cancer. *Journal of Clinical Oncology, 23*(15), 3629–3631.

Bor, R., Miller, R., Goldman, E., & Scher, I. (1993). The meaning of bad news in HIV disease counseling. *Psychology Quarterly, 6,* 69–80.

Browning, D., & Myer, E. C. (2003). Improving communication and strengthening relationships. In M. Z. Solomon, D. Browning, D. Dokken, A. Fleischman, W. Jose, K. H. Keller, et al. (Eds.), *The initiative for pediatric palliative care curriculum.* Newton MA: Education Development Center.

Chisholm, C., Pappas, D. J, & Sharp, M. C. (1997). Communicating bad news. *Obstetrics and Gynocology, 90,* 637–639.

Davey, H., Butow, P., & Armstrong, B. (2003). Cancer patient's preferences for written prognostic information provided outside the clinical context. *British Journal of Cancer, 89,* 7.

Davison, B. J., Parker, P. A., & Goldenberg, S. (2004). Patient's preferences for communicating a prostate cancer diagnosis and participating in medical decision-making. *British Journal of Urology, 93*, 47–51.

Friedman, H. S., & Silver, R. C. (Eds.) (2007). *Foundations of health psychology.* New York: Oxford University Press.

Fellows, D., Wilksinson, S., & Moore, P. (2003). Communication skills training for health care professionals working with cancer patients, their families and/or carers. *Cochrane Database Systematic Review,* (2), CD003751.

Halliwell, J., Mulcahy, P., Buetow, S., Bray, Y., Coster, G., & Osman, L. (2004). GP discussions of prognosis with patients with severe chronic obstructive pulmonary disease. *British Journal of General Practice, 54*(509), 904–908.

Krahn, G., Hallum, A., & Kime, C. (1993). Are there good ways to give "bad news"? *Pediatrics, 91,* 578–582.

Mack, J., & Grier, H. (2004). The day one talk. *Clinical Oncology, 22,* 563–566.

Rabow, M., & McPhee, S. (1999). Beyond breaking bad news. *Western Journal of Medicine, 171,* 260–263.

Sorensen, J., Rossel, P., & Holm, S. (2004). Patient-physician communication concerning participation in cancer chemotherapy. *British Journal of Cancer, 90,* 328–332.

Todd, W. E., & Ladon, E. H. (1998). Disease management: Maximizing treatment adherence and self-management. *Disease Management & Health Outcomes, 3,* 1–10.

Wolfe, J., Friebert, S., & Hilden, J. (2002). Caring for children with advanced cancer: Integrating palliative care. *Pediatric Clinics of North America, 49,* 1043–1062.

CHAPTER 7

Communications and Cultural Issues

Valerie A. Hart

It was Madeleine Leininger who introduced the concepts of transcultural care to nursing. She was interested in both the concepts of caring and the cultural aspects of nursing care (Leininger, 1985). Transcultural care has a holistic focus and is patient-centered while inviting clinicians to broaden their understanding of patients and families from different backgrounds. In today's rapidly changing demographic realities, the issues of cultural competence have risen to the top of relevant topics in health communication. Social structures identified by Leininger include religion (spirituality), kinship, politics, legal issues, education, economics, politics, philosophy, as well as gender, age, and values/beliefs. In order to fully understand a patient, these structures need to be understood and respected. For advanced practice nurses, a certification in Transcultural Nursing has been available since 1988 through the Transcultural Nursing Society. Recognizing the importance of attending to cultural issues, the American Association of Colleges of Nursing (AACN) has highlighted "cultural competence" in several of the outcome competencies in *The Essentials of Baccalaureate Nursing Education for Professional Nursing Practice* (AACN, 2008).

Culturally diverse patients present a variety of problems in a clinical setting, including symptom presentation as well as culturally determined meaning of an illness, which may include stigma (Kundhal & Kundhal, 2003). Cultural variations in the meaning of decision making and preferences for shared decision making require cultural sensitivity on the part of clinicians (Charles, Gafni, Whelan, & O'Brien, 2006). The clinical significance of cultural differences between patients and nurses has been identified (Lockhart & Resnick, 1997; Piette, Potter, & Heisler, 2003). In a study, Spanish-speaking diabetic patients treated in the outpatient department were more likely to report improved interpersonal interactions, leading to improved patient satisfaction when the physician spoke Spanish (Fernandez et al., 2004). In order to individualize care, the provider must

understand the patient's perception of health and illness, along with health practices, values, beliefs, and healthcare needs and decision-making preferences.
Becoming culturally competent is the mandate of both the novice as well as the
expert clinician. Both general communication and disease-specific communication have been shown to have an impact on self-management (Piette et al., 2003).

When people are ill and receiving health care, particularly in a hospital or clinic
setting, it seems that healthcare providers have the expectation that patients be
cooperative, undemanding, and respectful. This *good patient* role also includes not
asking too many questions, or challenging providers in regard to treatment decisions. In certain cultures, however, complaining and being demanding during a
bout of illness is rewarded, such as in Italian and American Jewish populations
(Andrews & Boyle, 1995). In contrast, Asian and Native American patients are
more likely to be quiet and compliant during illness. Appalachian patients may find
provider questions offensive due to the cultural value of not prying into others'
business or affairs. It is therefore important to consider what the cultural aspects
of the sick role may play a part with a patient or family who presents for care.

The National Center for Cultural Competence at Georgetown developed a
self-assessment for providers working in primary care. The tool, developed by
Cohen and Goode (1999), is available online at http://_www11.georgetown.edu/
research/gucchd/nccc. The assessment explores the physical environment and
materials provided for patients in an outpatient setting and clinician values and
attitudes. Questions related to specific clinical situations such as the birth of a
child with a disability, genetic disorders, and bereavement are included. In order
to gain cultural competence a provider must begin with a clear understanding of
their own background and cultural influences and biases. The process then requires a conscious and concerted effort on the part of the provider to learn about
different cultures and acknowledge one's personal responses to cultural differences. When working with a particular family or patient, this may mean including extended family members or friends in the treatment. There may be a need to
recognize and accept the presence of natural healers, such as shamans or curan-
deros. As with all patients and families, the clinician needs to identify the expectations regarding healthcare provision that are culturally based. Understanding the
traditions of a different culture related to gender may impact healthcare provision.
Knowing who is typically in charge of healthcare decisions for a family may be a
critical piece of information. Specific values related to authority, respect, and
control will be important to understand. The clinician also needs to keep in check
their reactions to differences that may grate on their own value system. Keeping
the patient and the family the center of the care is the requisite goal. In order to
provide culturally competent communication, the provider must engage in a program of self-awareness in regard to communication patterns and styles as well as
the social structures. In addition, the provider must examine aspects of cultural

phenomena including communication styles, time, space, and social organization (Giger & Davidhizar, 2004). Prejudice, bias, discrimination, and racism are a result of not understanding another's culture; stereotyping, judgment, and assignment of negative attributes to those who are different (Andrews & Boyle, 1995).

HEALTH INFORMATION LITERACY

The opposite of responding to patients with bias is the development of cultural sensitivity. In order to effectively communicate with any ethnic group the provider needs to familiarize themselves with the common cultural beliefs and values of the group, including beliefs associated with both health and illness. The clinician will need to apply this information to all aspects of patient care, from initial introduction through treatment and even termination of care. The problem of literacy presents a major problem when considering patient education. Barriers to health literacy can occur at the individual level, between providers and patients, and at the system level. Servellen (2009) notes that, although research abounds in the area of health education literacy, there is an erroneous assumption that the problem is written communications rather than the patient–provider relationship. The interventions of listening, pausing, and use of silence are particularly useful when working with patients with literacy issues. Indications that a patient possesses poor literacy related to health issues include: patients only asking questions after leaving the exam room; missed appointments; nonadherence; silence during visits; being accompanied by another adult who asks questions during the visit; and a patient who asks for information to be written down. Schillinger et al. (2003) have identified a method of communicating with low-literacy patients called "teach-back" or "loop." In this method the clinician asks the patient to restate whatever is communicated in order to ensure that miscommunications are not occurring. An additional benefit with this model is that patients may retain more information as a result of repeating instructions about medications or health-related facts. Clinicians are encouraged to avoid making the communication seem like a test of the patient, but instead view it as a test of how well the provider is able to communicate with the patient. A relaxed atmosphere that utilizes patience and reduces the patient's anxiety is optimal.

COMMUNICATIONS AND LATINO CULTURE

For purposes of example, the Latino or Hispanic culture will be examined, as it represents the fastest growing ethnic group in the United States. The dramatic increase in ethnic populations over the past several decades is reordering who we consider to be minorities in the United States. The continued growth specifically of the Latino or Hispanic population deserves special attention when considering health communication. There will be ever increasing demands for healthcare providers to better understand a cultural group whose distinct traditions and beliefs will place a lasting stamp on the healthcare system. Cora-Bramble and Williams (2000) distinguish between Hispanic and Latino in the following ways: *Latino* identifies those with ethnic origins from Spanish-speaking countries in Latin America as well as the Caribbean; *Hispanic* is a term created by the American government during the 1970s and later adopted by the US Census Bureau and includes those of Mexican, Puerto Rican, Cuban, and Central or South American culture, the common denominator being Spanish speaking. While the label *Latino* emphasizes geographic origin and history of those from Latin America, the term *Hispanic* is racially neutral. *Latinos* may prefer to be identified with their country of origin and some reject the label of *Hispanic*, as it intimates a connection with the country of Spain (Rodriguez, 1995). Minority groups experience high rates of cardiovascular disease, diabetes, asthma, and cancer due to various social determinants of health that may be outside the healthcare system (Betancourt, Green, Carrillo, & Ananeh-Firempong, 2003). For example, Latinos represent 13% of the US population but 25% lack health insurance, denying them often of preventative care, later stage diagnosis of conditions, and causing difficulty paying for prescribed medications (Andrulis,1998). In the 2000 US census, because of the "emerging sensitivities," the questions on race and Hispanic origin were revised. For purposes of the census, issues of race and Hispanic origin were seen as separate issues and separate questions were therefore included in the questionnaire. The question on Hispanic origin asked if respondents were *Spanish, Hispanic,* or *Latino.* The question on race asked what race the respondent considered themselves. Both questions were located in the self-identification portion of the form. The question of Hispanic origin preceded the question on race. In the 1990 census questionnaire the order was reversed and respondents had to choose one description, whereas in 2000 respondents could choose one or more. The report also used the terms *Hispanic* and *Latino* interchangeably. Because of these changes, the data on race is not directly comparable.

The 2000 census reported 35.3 million Hispanics, or 12.5% of the overall population of the United States. The prior census, in 1990, reported 23 million, or 9% of the population, which was a 53% increase from 1980. The Hispanic population has increased 57.9% since 1990 and, when the next census is taken in 2010, the numbers are expected to continue to increase in this population (Fig. 7-1). While it is unwise to generalize about any group, there is valuable information about cultural issues that can serve as guidelines for the clinician. Greater language proficiency has been shown to be associated with measures linked to a greater

Figure 7-1   Growth of Hispanic population in the United States, 1980 to 2000.

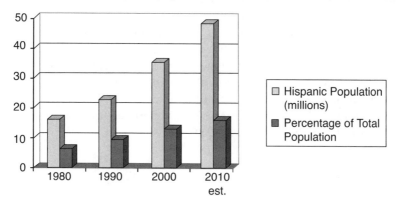

responsiveness to patients as well as behaviors leading to patient empowerment (Fernandez et al., 2004).

Another aspect of attempting to learn about another culture is the concept of *cultural dynamism*, or the fact that the changing needs of a population affect cultural realities. The larger society in which Latinos and Hispanics live affects shifting social norms. Among the themes that affect cross-cultural communication with Latinos, Cora-Bramble and Williams (2000) have identified:

Respect (*Respeto*)
Masculine Ideal (*Machismo*)
Family (*La Familia*)
Personal Relationships (*Personalismo*)

Respeto is the value of respect based on age, class, sex, and position. Men expect respect from women and children, and elders expect it from those younger than themselves. In addition, those in authority, including healthcare professionals, are accorded respect as a result of position.

Personalismo relates to warm and personal relationships. The cultural preference is in this direction, as opposed to neutral or chilly interactions. It is displayed by open affection upon greeting and gift-giving, even in professional settings and relationships.

Machismo refers to masculine strength and dignity. It has more of a relationship to honor than aggression. In the healthcare setting it may display itself by the male being the primary decision maker for other family members.

La Familia relates to the family as a highly valued social construct in the Latino community. The family extends far beyond the nuclear family and, in healthcare settings, will affect not only decision making but also involvement in actual treatment of a family member.

Taking into account these beliefs and values as aspects of healthcare, communication will need to be adjusted. For example, a series of closed-ended and direct questions could be viewed as unfriendly and abrasive or an indication of ignorance (Fishman, Bobo, Kosub, & Womeodu, 1993). The use of double negatives, a common habit of English-speaking health professionals (e.g., You don't want to . . . do you?), are difficult to understand and lead to misinformation and miscommunication in general (Mullavey-O'Byrne, 1994). Nonverbal communication messages also may take on different meanings to a Latino patient or family. Elements of nonverbal communication that tend to differ include (Cora-Bramble & Williams, 2000):

Gestures
Proximity
Touch
Eye contact
Expression of pain

Latino patients and families tend to utilize more gestures when describing a situation or symptom. They may need less physical distance between themselves and others when in a conversation or interaction, known as proximity. There may be more use of physical touching, which represents connection and involvement in a warm personal relationship. This may seem to contradict the fact that direct eye contact may be avoided, particularly with authority figures. In fact, direct and prolonged eye contact may be seen as a sign of disrespect on the part of the clinician. The way that pain is expressed in Latino culture can be characterized as more open and less repressed. Any of these differences from the cultural background of the healthcare provider may pose challenges and opportunities for personal growth. As with any cultural group, the clinician is wise to engage in further study of any ethnic or racial group that may comprise a portion of one's practice. Opportunities to interact with others who come from different background, in their setting and community, will teach invaluable lessons. The clinician needs to remain open and flexible while learning about a different culture.

USE OF INTERPRETERS

⚕ The role of interpreters is not simply to parrot what the patient is saying, but to serve as cultural liaison for the patient and family. In working with interpreters it is important to assess their familiarity with medical terms, symptoms, and diagnostic terminology. In a recent study of communication during clinician–family interactions, the findings are interesting when looking at the differences when interpreters were present (Thornton, Pham, Engelberg, Jackson, & Curtis, 2009).When interactions were not interpreted more verbal emotional support occurred. However, when interpreters were used, clinicians were less likely to allow pauses in the conversation and were also less likely to value family's questions or to demonstrate emotion. It would seem that utilizing the expertise of interpreters is more complicated than it might seem at first.

Andrews and Boyle (1995) offer a general guideline for nurses using an interpreter. When choosing an interpreter, the provider needs to know the language that the patient/family speaks in the home, as it may differ from what is spoken in public. It is advisable to avoid utilizing an interpreter from a rival tribe or region. Issues of choice of gender and class differences between patient and interpreter are also to be considered as they can affect the communication. Andrews and Boyle (1995) offers guidance when an interpreter is not available (Table 7-1):

Table 7-1   Interpreter Guidelines

When an Interpreter is present	When an interpreter is not available
Follow protocols involving introducing oneself as well as the interpreter to the patient and or family	Introduce yourself by stating your name, address the patient by their last name, and display warmth by eye contact and smiling
Avoid talking to the interpreter, but rather direct all communication to the patient and or family	Speak in an unhurried moderate voice; avoiding raising volume, which may be the tendency, in order to not frighten or startle the patient
Utilize culturally appropriate body language, including eye contact, gestures, etc., in order to facilitate the interaction	If the provider knows any words in the patient's language use them to communicate an awareness and respect for their culture
Only speak in a sentence or two at a time before allowing the interpreter to translate, and also ask the patient to respond slowly in small increments in order to assure accuracy of the communication	Use the simplest form of any word, avoiding medical jargon as well as slang

Table 7-1   Interpreter Guidelines   *(continued)*

When an Interpreter is present	When an interpreter is not available
Always ask the patient or family to repeat what it is that you have said in order to clarify and validate that the meaning of your words was accurately received	Avoid using pronouns; rather, refer to the patient by name when questioning about any behavior relevant to the visit
Expect to feel some frustration and allow for the added time that these interactions will require when scheduling for patient visits	Use pantomime for communicating simple words or actions
	Provide instructions in the proper sequence that the procedure is to be carried out
	Only discuss one topic at a time, and not in combinations
	Always have the patient validate what you are trying to communicate in order to check for accuracy

TRANSCULTURAL NURSING ASSESSMENT

The Andrews and Boyle Transcultural Nursing Assessment Guide is a tool which addresses cultural affiliations, values orientation, cultural sanctions and restrictions, health-related beliefs and practices, nutrition, socioeconomic considerations, religious affiliation, educational background, disease incidence, developmental considerations, and, of course, communication. In terms of communication the provider determines the following:

1. What languages are spoken and read both at home and in public?
2. What language does the patient and family prefer to communicate with you?
3. What is the patient's level of English fluency, both written and spoken?
4. Does the patient and family require an interpreter?
5. If an interpreter is needed, is it appropriate for this role to be filled by a family member?

6. Is there a specific request the patient has in regard to specific attributes of an interpreter, such as gender, age, etc.?
7. What are the linguistic norms and modes of communication?
8. Are there issues related to the patient's cultural background that require special considerations? This may include taboo topics, the norm of confidentiality.
9. What are the differences in regard to nonverbal communication with the patient and family?
10. How does this patient and family feel about having a provider who is from a different background?

ADDITIONAL CULTURAL MODELS

The University of Washington Medical Center has developed a series of tip sheets for clinicians, designed to increase awareness about patient preferences of patients from various cultures. Included in "Cultural–Clues" are Albanian, American Indian, Chinese, Korean, Russian, Latino, Somali, and Vietnamese. End-of-life care is defined for Russian, Latino, and Vietnamese patients and families.

The Cultural Clue for Somali patients notes that Somali patients are most likely "familiar with Western medical care for illness, but may be less familiar with well care, prenatal care, well child care or prevention" and so education in these areas is recommended. The role of preventive care, the role of the primary care team, and the process for getting a referral to a specialist are additional areas requiring education. The guideline goes on to discuss the fact that patients may have dietary requirements based on religious beliefs, such as a restriction from eating pork and the fact that family may bring food to the patient to ensure the proper diet is followed. It notes that the patient may use traditional remedies including prayer and herbal remedies such as habadsoda, a general healing herb, and that there is a belief that illness is caused by the evil eye; for example, not sharing food when you eat in front of a hungry person can cause stomach illness. It prompts the clinician to ask your patient what they believe is the reason for their illness. If appropriate, ask your patient if they need a visit from a holy person or sheikh. Under the category of "Helping Your Patient Understand Medications" is included the fact that patients expect an explanation for the illness, a medication, or some other form of treatment, and treatment options need to be explained while acknowledging the patient's symptoms. The clinician needs to be aware of the fact that patients fast from sunrise to sundown during the month of Ramadan, a holy month for Muslims, which occurs once a year and is based on the lunar calendar. It warns that the patient may only take medicines at night during this time and clinicians need to learn when Ramadan is celebrated each year and to alter medication choice or dosing to accommodate this practice. Under the category of "Understanding Childbearing Practices" it is noted that it is important for Somali women to be able to continue having children throughout their child-bearing years. Nutrition education needs to be included in giving prenatal care because malnutrition can be an issue, and the prenatal period provides an opportunity for families to learn about nutrition issues. Circumcision (infibulation) is an important issue to manage respectfully for Somali women. Clinicians are en-couraged to increase their familiarity with this procedure in order to gain deeper understanding as well as managing births for women who have had a circumci-sion. In regard to "How are medical decisions made in the Somali culture?" it is noted that often the father in the family has the role of the head of the household and decision maker; the mother is often the caregiver. Also, the male head of household may speak for the family because men were traditionally more edu-cated than women and may be more fluent in English, as well as affirming his role of being responsible for his family. To accommodate this it is advised that there be an interpreter present; confirm agreement with your female patients when necessary. In regard to treatment choices, it is noted that patients may be con-servative when making decisions about using new treatments or surgery because of a fear that aggressive treatments may cause more problems. Birth control and family planning are not widely practiced because of a preference to have large fam-ilies. Patients may want to avoid Caesarean sections because this procedure may limit the frequency of pregnancies. The informed consent process may be a new experience for Somali patients and, if this is your patient's first experience with informed consent, it requires explanation. An additional area of interest is that of "Gaining Family Support." In the Somali culture the entire extended family and friends may want to stay with the patient during their hospitalization. Clinicians need to be aware of the importance of this and consider how it can be accom-modated. Explain the visitation policy when the patient is admitted or before a surgery so that the patient/family know what to expect. Somali culture norms about touch, including social situations and modesty, are based on Islamic tradi-tions. It is advised that providers consider the modesty of women and girls when giving an exam. There is a strong preference for women to be seen by women healthcare workers and interpreters. Somali patients may prefer family members of the opposite gender leave the room during physical examination. It is advised that the provider find out if this is the case for your patient. Direct eye contact may be avoided because of modesty. A common greeting is to shake hands and say, "Salama Alaykum," which roughly translates, "May peace be with you." It is appropriate for men to shake hands only with men, and women with women. Adult women who follow traditional customs cover their bodies and veil their faces. If there is a male present during the exam, your patient may keep the veil on to maintain modesty. Additional information regarding cultural issues with this population is found on Ethnomed at http://ethnomed.org.

The *Physician's Practical Guide to Culturally Competent Care* is a self-directed training course for physicians and other healthcare professionals with a specific interest in cultural competency in the provision of care. To train physicians to care for diverse populations, the US Department of Health and Human Services' (HHS) Office of Minority Health (OMH) has commissioned the Cultural Competency Curriculum Modules (CCCM). These modules, encompassed in *A Physician's Practical Guide to Culturally Competent Care*, will equip physicians and other healthcare professionals with competencies that will enable them to better treat the increasingly diverse US population. This site, offering continuing medical education (CME) and continuing education units (CEU) credits, contains a variety of self-assessments, case studies, video vignettes, learning points, pre- and posttests, as well as the opportunity to submit your feedback and see what other participants think about the cases and content.

In a 2008 meta-analysis investigating the effectiveness of culturally appropriate diabetes health education on outcome measures for type 2 diabetes, researches found short-term effects on not only knowledge about diabetes and lifestyle, but also better glycemic control (Hawthorne, Robles, Cannings-John, & Edwards, 2008). In addition, the researchers cited a need for long-term studies that compare various types of culturally appropriate health education within defined ethnic minority groups in order to advance this area of knowledge.

A useful approach when attempting to increase cultural competence in clinicians is to regard the patient as teacher in terms of cultural and social issues. It is the patient who can best inform healthcare providers about different styles of communication, family roles, gender issues, and decision-making preferences. Betancourt et al. (2003) identifies the barriers to culturally competent care as:

Lack of diversity in the healthcare workforce
Lack of diversity in healthcare leadership
Poorly designed systems of care
Problematic communication between providers and patients of different
    ethnic and racial backgrounds

In order to address these barriers, the following recommendations are offered in a 2002 field report (Betancourt et al., 2003):

Establishment of programs for minority healthcare leadership development
Hire and promote minorities in health care

Conduct community assessments

Establish feedback mechanisms in regard to patient racial, ethnic, and language preference

Develop quality measures for diverse patient populations

Ensure linguistically appropriate health education materials

Have on-site interpreter services

Develop health information that is written at the appropriate literacy level and is targeted to the language and cultural norms of specific patient populations

Use research tools to detect errors due to lack of cultural competence such as language barriers

Develop standards for measuring cultural competence

Collect race, ethnic, and language preference data from patients

Milton Bennett (1993) has developed a model of cultural sensitivity as well as an assessment tool to measure an individual's level of cultural sensitivity, the Intercultural Developmental Inventory (IDI). This model utilizes a developmental approach which includes six stages:

1. Denial of differences
2. Defense against differences
3. Minimization of differences
4. Acceptance of differences, or new awareness
5. Adaptation, or a new way of behaving
6. Integration of cultural differences

As with most developmental models, the stages are fluid and individuals may advance or regress along the way toward the ultimate stage of integration.

Kleinman and Benson (2006) have introduced a broader perspective from that of cultural competence. They argue that, in medicine, the notion of cultural competence has been reduced to technical skills based on only ethnicity, nationality, and language. Instead of stereotyping patients or applying cultural factors that may not be central to the health issue being addressed, these authors offer an alternative definition of culture. This definition includes a dynamic understanding of culture and includes economic, religious, political, biological, and psychological realities. They view culture as a "process" which affects emotional and moral meaning for the individual. Utilizing this broader view of culture allows the clinician to include not only religious practices but also the meaning of interpersonal attachments. It acknowledges the fact that, within the same ethnic group, there exist wide differences. Therefore the patient's age, gender, political association, class, religion, and personality need to be considered. The clinician adopting this framework attends to understanding the patient's experiences as he/she does; in other words, applies the concepts of empathy. Utilizing *miniethnogrophy* as an approach the clinician follows a series of steps:

1. Identify ethnic identity and determine its relevance for the patient by asking the patient specifically the connection of ethnicity and illness.
2. Evaluate what is at stake for the patient and family. Aspects may include intimate relationships, finances, and spiritual considerations.
3. Formulate an understanding of an illness narrative as explained by the patient and family. In other words, what is the meaning of the illness for the patient and family?
4. Evaluate both stressors and support systems, including living arrangements, work, finances, relationships, etc.
5. Examine the influence of culture on the patient–provider relationship. This step includes self-reflection on the part of the clinician and honestly facing bias and stereotyping.
6. Examine efficacy of using a cultural framework with the patient and family. This includes identifying side effects of the approach, which may include an overemphasis on culture or intrusiveness for the patient and family (Kleinman & Benson, 2006).

COMMUNICATION EXERCISES

1. Cultural Awareness

Pair off as patient and provider: 30 minutes.

Provider:

Conduct an assessment of this patient.

Patient:

Compose a patient profile that represents being from another culture and develop a symptom presentation, making your cultural background a component of your concerns.

Discussion:

Share with one another the issues that were raised during the interaction.

Discuss any miscommunication that occurred as a result of cultural differences.

Switch roles and repeat.

_____

_____

_____

_____

_____

_____

_____

_____

2. Cultural Competence

Pair off as patient and provider: 30 minutes.

Provider:

Respond to your patient, keeping in mind that you do not share the same cultural background. Utilize your skills in cultural competence to understand this patient's concerns as well as to communicate whatever information you need to about their condition.

Patient:

Develop a clinical scenario based on the fact that you have socioculturally based health beliefs and medical practices, including home remedies.

Discussion:

Share your experiences with one another as patient and provider.

What were the difficult aspects or frustrations for each of you?

What aspects were easier than you expected?

Share with each other any experiences you have had with similar patients in a clinical setting.

How could this exercise inform your practice?

Are there implications for professional development?

What recommendations do you each have for a more effective interaction?

Switch roles and repeat.

_____

_____

_____

_____

_____

_____

_____

_____

3. Culturally Sensitive Interview

Pair off as patient and provider: 30 minutes.

Provider:

You are aware that your patient is from another culture and for whom English is a second language. There is no interpreter available, and your patient has a rudimentary level of speaking and understanding English. Conduct your interview with these issues in mind.

Patient:

Present to your primary care provider displaying a different style of communication, decision-making preference, family role, and general mistrust of healthcare professionals.

Discussion:

Share the perspective of both patient and provider with one another.

Where there any communication blocks during the interview?

How were misconceptions or possible miscommunications handled by the provider?

Provider:

When did you conclude that the patient has issues of trust where you were concerned?

How did this manifest itself?

What was your reaction to this conclusion?

What strategies did you employ to deal with the lack of trust in healthcare professionals?

Discuss how effective these strategies were from your perspective.

How did you react to other differences such as roles, decision-making preferences, etc., of this patient?

Assess your cultural sensitivity in this interaction.

Patient:

How would you assess the provider's response to your different views, decision-making preferences, and roles?

How did this color your satisfaction with the encounter?

Would you be interested in returning to see this provider based on this interaction? If yes, why? And if no, why not?

What did you determine was difficult for your provider?

What do you base this on?

Ask your provider if your assumption is correct.

Discussion:

What have you each learned from this interaction?

Did the exercise highlight issues related to cultural competence and sensitivity for you?

Have your experiences in a clinical setting mirror this interaction? In what way?

Switch roles and repeat.

_____

_____

_____

_____

_____

_____

_____

_____

4. Somali Culture

Pair off as patient and provider: 30 minutes.

Provider:

Your goal for this interaction is to educate your patient about the importance of preventative care, in this case, prenatal care. Conduct the consultation with this goal in mind.

Patient:

You are from Somalia and recently emigrated to the United States. You are present because of a question of being pregnant. Because of your culture, you are not familiar with the concept of prenatal care.

Discussion:

Patient, assess how your provider dealt with the educational component of your visit.

Did your clinician introduce themselves, including an explanation of their clinical role?

Did your clinician share their experience in caring for similar patients?

How did your provider handle the differences in your understanding of preventative health care?

Did your clinician ask about dietary restrictions based on religious beliefs during the interview?

Did your clinician inquire about herbal remedies?

Did your clinician ask you what your perspective on pregnancy is?

Provider, discuss your experience of conducting the clinical consultation. What aspects were difficult? Why?

Did you find yourself frustrated at any point in the interview?

What were the biggest challenges for you as a clinician?

What ideas do you have about improving your competence when working with this population?

Share your experiences with this population, both on a personal and professional level.

_____

_____

_____

_____

_____

_____

_____

_____

5. American Indian Culture

Pair off as patient and provider: 30 minutes.

Provider:

Conduct an initial assessment of this patient.

Patient:

You have been having stomach pain for about 1 month. Because of your cultural heritage you have been taught to resist any expression of pain, so you report feeling "uncomfortable" instead. Your history has also made you leery of traditional institutions, including health care. You arrive 20 minutes late for your appointment, as is accepted in your culture.

Discussion:

Provider, how did you proceed when you experienced resistance to openly discuss pain with this patient?

Did you have an understanding of your patient's lateness based on cultural awareness of differences?

Did you use storytelling as a strategy?

Did you remember to avoid eye contact with this patient?

What strategies did you employ in order to build trust with this patient?

If your interview involved any touching of the patient, how did you manage this aspect of the interaction?

If the patient was wearing jewelry or hair ornaments that needed to be removed for the exam, how did you manage this?

Overall, how comfortable were you during this interview?

What might have improved your comfort or feelings of competence in future?

Patient, assess the ability of your provider to honor your cultural differences.

Did your clinician ask permission to touch you before doing so?

If you were wearing jewelry with spiritual meaning for you, how did your provider manage this aspect of the interview?

Discuss what your provider did and did not do in regard to establishing trust during the interaction.

Switch roles and repeat.

JOURNALING EXERCISES

1. Cultural Competency

How do you assess your ability to be culturally sensitive in a patient encounter?

Describe an encounter with a patient from a different culture that was frustrating and/or disappointing to you.

Describe an encounter with a patient from a different culture that was highly satisfying to you.

What do you think was significantly different about these two clinical encounters?

_____

_____

_____

_____

_____

_____

_____

_____

2. Cultural Competency

Identify the cultural biases that you are aware of. What are the sources of these ideas and feelings?

How might these ideas/beliefs interfere with your ability to provide patient care?

How might these ideas/beliefs enhance your ability to provide patient care?

How might you develop a plan to address the obstacles that may exist in this area for you?

_____

_____

_____

_____

_____

_____

_____

_____

3. Cultural Competency

Describe a situation in which you would request the presence of an interpreter in a clinical encounter.

If you have worked with an interpreter in the past, describe the experience.

If you have not had the experience of working with an interpreter, what do you imagine would be the challenges?

What would be your goals when requesting the presence of an interpreter in a clinical encounter?

_____

_____

_____

_____

_____

_____

_____

_____

REFERENCES

American Association of Colleges of Nursing. (2008). *The essentials of baccalaureate nursing education for professional nursing practice*. Washington, DC: AACN.

Andrews, M., & Boyle, J. (1995). *Transcultural concepts in nursing care* (Vol. 2). Philadelphia: J. B. Lippincott Co.

Andrulis, D. P. (1998). Access to care is the centerpiece in the elimination of socioeconomic disparities in health. *Annals of Internal Medicine, 129*, 12–16.

Bennett, M. J. (1993). Towards ethnorelativism: A development model of intercultural sensitivity. In R. M. Paige (Ed.), *Education for the Intercultural Experience* (pp. 27–71). Yarmouth, ME: Intercultural Press.

Betancourt, J. R., Green, A. R., Carrillo, J. E., & Ananeh-Firepong, O. (2003). Defining cultural competence: A practical framework for addressing racial/ethnic disparities in health and health care. *Public Health* Reports, *118*, 293–301.

Charles, C., Gafni, A., Whelan, T., & O'Brien, M. A. (2006). Cultural influences on the physician-patient encounter: The case of shared treatment decision-making. *Patient Education and Counseling, 63*(3), 262–267.

Cohen, E., & Goode, T. D. (1999). *Rationale for cultural competence in primary health care*. Washington, DC: National Center for Cultural.

Cora-Bramble, D., & Williams, L. (2000). Explaining illness to Latinos: Cultural foundations and messages. In B. B. Whaley (Ed.), *Explaining illness: Research, theory, and strategies* (pp. 257–281). Mahwah, NJ: Lawrence-Erlbaum and Associates.

Fernandez, A., Schillinger, D., Grumbach, K., Rosenthal, A., Stewart, A., Wang, F., et al. (2004). Physician language ability and cultural competence. *Journal of General Internal Medicine, 19,* 167–174.

Fishman, B. M., Bobo, L., Kosub, K., & Womeodu, R. J. (1993). Cultural issues in serving minority populations. *American Journal of Medical Sciences, 306*(3), 160–166.

Giger, J. N., & Davidhizar, R. E. (2004). *Transcultural nursing: Assessment and Intervention.* St. Louis: CV Mosby.

Hawthorne, K., Robles,Y., Cannings-John, R., & Edwards, A.G. (2008). Culturally appropriate health education for type 2 diabetes mellitus in ethnic minority groups. *Cochrane Database of Systematic Reviews,* (3), CD006424.

Kleinman, A., & Benson, P. (2006). Anthropology in the clinic: The problem of cultural competency and how to fix it. *PLoS Medicine, 3*(10), e294.

Kundhal, K. K., & Kundhal, P. S. (2003). Cultural diversity: An evolving challenge to physician-patient communication. *Journal of the American Medical Association, 289,* 94.

Leininger, M. (1985). Transcultural diversity and universality: A theory of nursing. *Nursing and Health Care, 6,* 208–212.

Lockhart, J., & Resnick, L. (1997). Teaching cultural competence. *Nurse Educator, 22,* 27–31.

Mullavey-O'Byrne, C. (1994). Intercultural communication for health care professional. In R.Y. Brislin (Ed.), *Improving intercultural interactions* (pp. 171–196). Thousand Oaks, CA: Sage.

Piette, J., Potter, D. S., & Heisler, M. (2003). Dimensions of patient-provider communication and diabetes self-care in an ethnically-diverse patient population. *Journal of General Internal Medicine, 18,* 624–633.

Rodriguez, S. (1995). *Hispanics in the United States: An insight into group characteristics.* Washington, DC: Department of Health and Human Service.

Schillinger, D., Piette, J., Grumbach, K., Wang, F., Wilson, C., Daher, C., Leong-Grotz, K., et al. (2003). Closing the loop: Physician communication with diabetic patients who have low health literacy. *Archives of Internal Medicine, 16*(3), 7.

Servellen, G. (2009). *Communication skills for the health care professional.* Sudbury, MA: Jones and Bartlett.

Thornton, J. D., Pham, K., Engelberg, R. A., Jackson, J. C., & Curtis, J. R. (2009). Families with limited English proficiency receive less information and support in interpreted intensive care unit family conferences. *Critical Care Medicine, 37,* 89–95.

CHAPTER 8

Interdisciplinary and Peer Communication

Ann M. McPhee

*Coming together is a beginning. Keeping together is progress.
Working together is success.*

—Henry Ford

The importance of quality communication in health care cannot be understated. A breakdown in communication can have devastating effects on patient outcomes. The literature suggests that barriers to communication exist between healthcare providers. I contend that barriers do exist but progress has been made to improve communication and reduce the inherent conflict between providers.

Today's healthcare team faces additional challenges that include the slumping economy, inadequate labor pool, poor staffing, cost containment, limited resources, and downsizing. Although conflict has been identified as a fundamental problem of organizational life, conflict among healthcare professionals is detrimental to patients and team performance (Cox, 2001; Valentine, 1995).

HORIZONTAL VIOLENCE

An added concern for nurses and nurse practitioners is the presence of horizontal violence in the workplace. Horizontal violence is hostile and aggressive behavior by individual or group members toward another member or group members of the larger group (Duffy, 1995). The notion that "nurses eat their young" is not a new one, but one that is extremely disturbing in a profession where the nurse is viewed as caring and compassionate. Nurse-to-nurse, or horizontal violence, can manifest in many forms including verbal abuse, gossip, scapegoating, criticism, sabotage, or refusing to behave in a cooperative and respectful manner on the job. It is the opposite of being a team player, or simply being a kind human being to your colleagues. Mocking another, withholding information, blaming, humiliating another, breaking confidentiality, and behaving in an elitist manner are all behaviors that fall into this category.

Unfortunately, horizontal violence is seen globally. The International Council of Nurses (ICN), in a guideline on the issue, noted that worldwide nurses are three times more likely to experience violence in the workplace, among all service occupations (ICN, 2004). Attempts to try to understand horizontal violence include knowledge concerning oppressed group behavior. Paulo Freire, a Brazilian educator and philosopher, wrote *Pedagogy of the Oppressed* (1972), which attempts to explain why groups who have experienced oppression so often become oppressors themselves. Freire warns that the violence of the oppressors "prevents the oppressed from being fully human" and because oppressors dehumanize and violate rights they also become dehumanized. He discussed the "oppressor–oppressed contradiction." One would think that if one had experienced oppression it would lead to more compassionate treatment of others, when just the reverse is true.

Effects of Horizontal Violence

Wilkie (1996) has outlined the progression of the effects of horizontal violence.

Stage 1: activation of the flight or fight response. During this stage, people experience decreased self-esteem, anxiety, sleep disturbances, and low morale.

Stage 2: sleep deprivation and neurotransmitter depletion. People experience difficulty with motivation, emotional control, and may have physical manifestations such as hypertension.

Stage 3: brain circuit breakers are activated. There is a decreased tolerance for sensory stimulation, depression, and disconnection, leading to disturbed personal relationships and a need to withdraw from the workplace.

The Joint Commission (2007) has identified that unresolved conflict and disruptive behavior adversely affect safety and quality of care. The Center for American Nurses, a professional association dedicated to professional support for nurses, has developed a position paper, Lateral Violence and Bullying in the Workplace, which not only defines both types of behaviors but also call for a "cultural change" and links the issue to retention of nurses in the workplace. Most nurses have experienced some form of horizontal violence at different points in their careers. The presentation may be in the form of criticism, bullying, passive aggression, or as simple as a peer withholding information about a patient. This form of violence perpetuates the nurse's lack of collegiality and contributes to the reduced professional status as compared with that of medicine (Baltimore, 2006).

In the nursing profession, explanations for horizontal violence have, in the main, been influenced by oppression and feminist theories. Roberts (1983) suggests that intra-staff conflict in nursing is characteristic of their oppressed status. Other theorists suggest that the conflict between nurses is not unique to the profession but more the norm in women's relationships. Historically, the profession has been dominated by women, thus setting the stage for conflict between nurses and, ultimately, a barrier between the nurse and physician collaboration.

Nurse and physician miscommunication represents gender differences at work that may represent the inherent imbalance in power relations between men and women (Farrell, 2001). The physician oftentimes views the nurse as a subservient partner in health care. Referred to as "my nurse," the physician dictates orders that the nurse carries out with little or no questioning of authority. The nurse may not have the knowledge or the skill to challenge the decision making of the physician.

It was not so long ago that a nurse would stand and offer her seat when the physician entered the room. This is a good example of how men have traditionally exercised power over women, thereby placing women in inferior and vulnerable positions relative to men. Nursing is seen as case and point (Davies & Hughes, 1995).

Where does the nurse practitioner fit into this equation? Most nurse practitioners have practiced at the bedside, aligned with other staff nurses, prior to completing their advanced practice education. They have often come up through the ranks and encountered the same power struggles as their peers. As they enter into their new role, where they are able to diagnose and treat patients, the dynamic between the physician and nurse practitioner changes.

It is important to remember that nurse practitioner role evolved in the mid-1960s at a time when it was difficult to bring health care to remote areas. The patient populations included impoverished communities, the urban uninsured, and rural communities where access to a provider could be hours away.

COLLABORATION AND TEAMWORK

A committee formed by Secretary of the Department of Health, Education, and Welfare (DHEW) reported in the *Journal of the American Medical Association* (DHEW Secretary's Committee to Study Extended Roles for Nurses, 1972) that the new role for nursing "affords an opportunity for significant and necessary extension of the part that nurses play in making health care accessible to a population whose demands and expectation impose an increasingly heavy burden on the present healthcare delivery system" (p. 1232). Partnering with physicians improves access to care as well as bringing nursing's focus on holistic healthcare into the plan of care for the patient. The partnership is a cost effective, efficient way of bringing healthcare services to patients, no matter the setting.

Unlike physician assistants, the nurse practitioner is capable of working independently and interdependently with members of the healthcare team. Nurse practitioners are highly skilled at managing acute and chronic disease processes, including conditions such as diabetes and hypertension. They also bring a focus on health promotion and disease prevention through patient education and collaboration with the patient and family. The contribution that the nurse practitioner brings to health care is another reason why communication is so important when interacting with the team and the patient and family.

In spite of the value that the nurse practitioner brings to the healthcare arena, the role continues to be controversial in the eyes of many of our physician colleagues due in part to lack of understanding of the role and the nurse practitioner's scope of practice. The American College of Physicians (ACP) recently released a policy monograph stating that, "in the patient-centered medical home (PCMH) model, care for patients is best served by a multidisciplinary team where the clinical team is led by a physician" (ACP, 2009, p. 2).

Today, most nurse practitioners hold a master's degree in their respective specialty. The inconsistencies in educational preparation that existed early on have been replaced with core curriculums that are more consistent with the nurse practitioner's scope of practice. In a bold move, the American Association of Colleges of Nursing (AACN) issued a position statement which called for the Doctor of Nursing Practice (DNP) as the terminal degree for advanced practice nursing by 2015. Unlike the traditional PhD, which is research based, the DNP is a practice-focused degree. AACN cited a changing healthcare environment that demanded a higher level of preparation for advanced practice nurses, which include nurse practitioners, clinical specialists, nurse midwives, and nurse anesthetists. The DNP movement has not been without its critics inside nursing (Carlson, 2003; Chase & Pruitt, 2006; Dracup, & Bryan-Brown, 2005). While some called for constructive debate (Broome, 2005; Fulton & Lyon, 2005), others explored the impact on other health professions (Clement, 2005) and there has been clear disagreement with the degree (Meleis & Dracup, 2005).

In 2008, changes to Resolution 214 attempted to impose physician supervision of DNP practice, although nurse practitioners had autonomous and independent practices in 22 states at the time. The American Nurses Association (ANA) responded to the amendment by noting that all matters pertaining to nurse's scope of practice are handled by state boards of nursing, state legislatures, and nursing itself (ANA, 2008). The ANA reminded the American Medical Association (AMA) that, in an effort to respond to a changing healthcare environment, flexibility and cooperation between nurses and physicians was required. In 2006 the AMA vigorously debated a resolution, introduced by the Georgia delegate, denouncing the use of the term *doctor* for the DNP at a Delegates meeting in Chicago, regardless of the fact that a doctorate in any field entitles the successful candidate to adopt the term. This resolution was defeated. The current policy monograph of the ACP (2009) states:

> *Questions have been raised about the adequacy of NP training and certification, comparisons drawn by NPs to the care delivered by physicians, quality of patient outcomes, and perceived intentions to displace or replace primary care physicians (p. 4) and in regard to the DNP:*

> *The use of the prefix "Dr." or "Doctor" by NPs who have completed the DNP degree could lead to confusion and misconceptions by patients (p.9).*

The Coalition for Patient's Rights (CPR), formed in 2006, is an organization, consisting of 37 organizations, whose mission is to counter AMA efforts to scale back the scope of practice for advanced practice nurses. The organization views its mandate in terms of protecting patient's choice of healthcare providers. The AMA's Scope of Practice Partnership, formed in 2006, specifically cited the DNP among its concerns, arguing that the public would be confused by titling between doctorally prepared nurses and physicians. Other health disciplines were also targeted, including limiting licensure, limiting independent practitioners such as doctors of chiropractic, acupuncturists, and naturopathic physicians.

Despite its critics, development of DNP programs has experienced explosive growth and now more than 80 programs are currently accepting students. A consensus model addressing issues related to regulation, licensure, accreditation, certification, and education was developed by a total of 41 nursing organizations reaching consensus (APRN Joint Dialogue Group Report, 2008). The report notes 2015 as the year by which full implementation will be achieved. *Essentials of Doctoral Education for Advanced Nursing Practice*, developed by AACN (2006), has identified "Interprofessional Collaboration for Improving Patient and Population Health Outcomes" as one of the essentials for the DNP. Included in this essential is the expectation that DNP programs prepare graduates to "employ effective communication and collaborative skills in the development and implementation of practice models, peer review, practice guidelines, health policy, standards of care, and/or other scholarly products; lead interprofessional teams in the analysis of complex practice and organizational issues; employ consultative and leadership skills with intraprofessional and interprofessional teams to create change in health care and complex healthcare delivery systems" (ANCC, 2006, p. 14). There is a clear mandate for the advanced practice nurse of the future to take a leadership role and to work in a collaborative fashion with other professionals. Nurse practitioners still have a long way to go to reverse the physician's view of the nurse practitioner as a "physician extender." Unfortunately, this view undermines the value that the nurse and the profession of nursing bring to patient- and family-centered care. We cannot lose sight of the fact that the nurse practitioner role was never meant to replace the physician role but, instead, to augment patient care while expanding the role of the professional nurse. The importance of building strong nurse practitioner and physician partnerships lends itself to positive working relationships where collaborative practice bonds are formed. Once again, the value of communication between disciplines cannot be overlooked as it is the only way that improved understanding of roles will be achieved.

In 2001, the Institute of Medicine (IOM) published *Crossing the Quality Chasm: A New Health System for the 21st Century.* The publication stressed need for change in the American healthcare system, stressing a new approach to meet the needs of patients and their families. They produced a series of rules that, if implemented, would redesign and improve health care. For the purposes of this chapter, we will focus on the 10th rule, where enhanced cooperation among clinicians was identified. The IOM stressed that the existing healthcare system in the United States protects professional prerogatives and separate roles. The current system shows too little cooperation and teamwork. Patients suffer through lost continuity, redundancy, excess costs, and miscommunication (IOM, 2001, p. 83). The IOM further states that excessive emphasis is placed on individual credentials rather than approaching the care that is needed to complete the task at hand.

There are increasingly more male nurses and women physicians in the workplace. The shift has been positive for all professions and the healthcare system as a whole, as the playing field for providers is less patriarchal. Providers, regardless of gender, come to the table with expertise, knowledge, and a voice to advocate for patients and their families. Each discipline has the capacity to bring strengths that help the patient and family set goals that are reasonable and attainable. We would be remiss if we did not point out that it takes an entire team to execute the patient's plan of care. Therefore we cannot underestimate the contributions of all team members including the physician, nurse practitioner, nurse, social worker, dietician, physical therapist, and other disciplines in promoting safe patient- and family-centered care.

In primary care, we look to the primary care provider (physician and/or nurse practitioner) to be the gate keeper who coordinates services needed for the patient. The balance between disciplines promotes a win–win situation for the patient and the family. Physicians are highly skilled at focusing on objective data, including the patient's physical assessment and diagnostic studies, to establish a differential diagnosis. Once a diagnosis is established and a plan of care is put in place, the reality of the patient's ability to follow the plan comes into play. The nurse practitioner, although able to diagnose and treat the patient, places an emphasis on the broader picture where consideration is given to the patient's psychosocial situation, including cultural barriers, education, income, family support systems, and living situation. The partnership promotes improved patient outcomes and improved patient and family satisfaction.

In order to achieve strong collaborative practices, the team must share common goals and a commitment to reach positive outcomes for the patient and the family. All providers must respect and value the individual contributions that each individual brings to the table. Shared responsibility in the decision making is the key component in executing a healthcare plan. There needs to be a shift between professional relationships to improve and enhance care. The healthcare team needs to focus on having the right person doing the right job, at the right time (Nelson, Batalden, & Godfrey, 2007).

Effective teams must be created, nurtured, and maintained. There must be an understanding that team members are typically trained in separate disciplines and educational programs. Members of the team may not appreciate each other's strengths or recognize weaknesses except in crises, and they may not have been trained together to use established or new technologies (IOM, 2001, p. 131). Respect and trust are built over time as comfort levels between providers expand and grow.

Effective communication is essential in order to build positive working relationships and is a critical component in team building.

Considerable research has gone into identifying the characteristics of effective teams (Fried, Topping, & Rundall, 2000; see Box 8-1). Effective teams have

---

Box 8-1   Characteristics of Effective Teams

Team makeup, such as having appropriate size and composition and the ability to reduce negative effects of status differences between physicians and nurses
Team processes, such as communication structures, conflict management, and leadership that emphasizes excellence and conveys clear goals and expectations
The nature of the team's tasks, such as matching roles and training to the level of complexity and promoting cohesiveness when work is highly interdependent
The environmental context, such as obtaining needed resources and establishing appropriate rewards

a culture that fosters openness, collaboration, teamwork, and learning from mistakes (IOM, 2001, p. 132).

Interdisciplinary rounds are an effectual tool to develop and strengthen patient goals. Remembering to include the patient and family in rounds will optimize the patient outcomes.

In terms of team processes, the introduction of "huddles" related to patient care needs and work demands can be powerful. The concept of huddling is not new. Huddles are common in sports and are regularly used by teams to evaluate how the game is going and whether there needs to be a change in strategy (Shermont et al., 2008). In health care, the huddle is an effective way to evaluate care demand, patient acuity, and stress levels of providers. Interdisciplinary huddles also promote positive working relationships. Individuals get to know each other's strengths, weaknesses, and ways of communicating. In the end, the right person becomes responsible for the right job, at the right time, given the understanding of what components of the plan the patient and family are capable to follow. Over time, the huddle will remove barriers in the hierarchical strata by helping team members value the contributions that each member, including the patient, brings to the table. Additional benefits can be measured in improved communication, decreased work stress, and increased opportunities for teaching, planning the day's work, adjusting the schedules, and thinking ahead to meet patient's needs while improving efficiency (Nelson et al., 2007, p. 145).

CONFLICT

Even in the best relationships, conflict between individuals is inevitable due to a breakdown in communication. In the face of conflict, it is important to walk away from the situation, regroup (within 24 hours or more), and return later to identify and confront the root cause of the issue. Many times, the root cause of the issue is a symptom of a suboptimal workflow or system, not the individual provider involved in the conflict. The distancing from the situation provides an opportunity for each individual to take the emotion out of the ensuing interaction and focus on the true reason for the initial confrontation. The individuals involved then meet and come to consensus about the issue and put the conflict behind them. Individuals must be willing to share candid, honest feedback with their peers regarding the concern. Optimally there will be a change in personal behavior, policy, or workflow to promote a better patient outcome.

Strategies to reduce and minimize conflict within an interdisciplinary team include one or all of the following (Julia & Thompson, 1994):

- Built-in process to review decisions, including review and definition of goals, the direction of the team, and priorities

- Role clarification through the discussion of such topics and knowledge base, professional stereotypes, specializations, autonomy, competencies, responsibilities, and codes of ethics
- Examination of overlapping roles and renegotiation of role assignments
- Recognition of professional hierarchies and discussion of their impact on team functioning (status and delegation of authority issues are a part of this activity)
- Opportunities for improving interprofessional skills of team members teaching processes of handling conflict

Team members learn to rely on the strengths of each other. Inherent in improved communication, conflict becomes manageable resulting in the patient and family benefiting from the provider's ability to challenge the issue, remove the emotion the provider is feeling, and focus on the best outcome for the patient. Team members are able to acknowledge the important contributions that all parties bring to the plan of care.

Fitzgerald, Millonowicz, and Leslie (2008) defined communication as the key tool that healthcare professionals must use to elicit cooperation among individuals in the delivery of healthcare services. It is an integral part of social-ization and imperative in establishing relationships. This holds true for the entire healthcare team, including the patient and family, where evidence-based prac-tice and patient-centered care may clash.

Many patients have become informed consumers of health care due to the increased availability of healthcare information through the Internet and other sources. Patients will challenge treatment options after completing their own research, expect to have a voice in treatment decision making, and demand greater accountability from their providers when assisting them in reaching their goals. This is a good thing, because the patient can voice what is reasonable for them and help the team understand what their values, needs, and expectations related to treatment options.

HEALTH OUTCOMES

The IOM (2001) highlighted the importance of evidence-based care and positive health outcomes in its definition of quality of care as, "the degree to which health services for individuals and populations increase the likelihood of desired of desired health outcomes and are consistent with current professional knowledge." Quality primary care is measured by positive patient outcomes in response to evidence-based health care in the 21st century, including the safety, effectiveness, timeliness, efficiency, equitability, and patient centeredness of care (IOM, 2001). The IOM initiatives are supported by nursing practice standards, which highlight the importance of patient-centered approaches to achieving quality health care (ANA, 2004).

Evidence-based medicine strives to improve patient outcomes through the standardization of medical care by incorporating the use of protocols and guidelines into the patient's plan. The "best practice" model may enhance quality, but the "cookbook" approach to patient care oftentimes leaves little room for the integration of individual provider clinical expertise or patient preference. Evidence-based medicine has responded to this criticism with language that encourages the integration of guidelines, protocols, and best practices along with clinical expertise and patient preferences into decision making (Sackett, Rosenberg, Gray, Haynes, & Richardson, 1996).

The patient-centered care model frames "disease within the context of the patients' lives and experiences and does not view patients as purely biomedical entities" (Dawood, 2005, p. 22). Patient-centered care is not a new concept for the nurse practitioner; holistic approaches to patient care have been a core component of nursing practice for many years.

A criticism of the patient-centered care model relates to the additional time that it takes to gather pertinent information from the patient, thus decreasing provider productivity. It is important to remember that providers cannot afford to *not* invest this time because the patient's ability to follow the plan of care may be determined through this type of interviewing.

In the end, positive patient outcomes are directly related to everyone's ability to find the balance between evidence-based medicine and patient-centered care. Team work, positive relationships, enhanced communication, and mutual respect by everyone involved are key components when measuring the success of interdisciplinary interactions.

COMMUNICATION EXERCISES

1. Interdisciplinary and Peer Communication

Pair off as nurse practitioner and registered nurse.

Registered Nurse:

You arrive on a busy surgical unit to make rounds on your patients. During a chart review, you note that Mrs. Janesfield has a dangerously low potassium level that was not reported to your team. You have a history of working with the nurse caring for the patient and have found that she oftentimes overlooks important ancillary test reports.

Nurse Practitioner:

You proceed to the patient's room to complete your physical assessment of the patient before ordering additional diagnostic studies and the needed supplement of potassium. You are frustrated with your perceived lack of accountability by the nurse and want to confront this nurse with your findings.

Do a second assessment of the patient, including the nurse and hospitalist physician at the patient's bedside. Establish your plan of care for this patient based on your clinical findings after including the patient and team members in your discussion.

Discussion:

Identify the strengths and weaknesses of both of these approaches when assessing the patient.

How were both approaches different?

Identify the best approach for you, the nurse practitioner, to address your concerns about the nurse's performance.

Identify the possible reasons for the nurse to have missed the critical lab results.

Share with one another examples of real life scenarios that you have been involved in when caring for patients.

What worked and what did not?

_____

_____

_____

_____

_____

_____

2. Interdisciplinary and Peer Communication

Pair off as nurse practitioner and physician.

The scenario is that you, the nurse practitioner, need to consult with a physician in your practice regarding the clinical findings you have identified when examining Mr. Smith. You are immediately challenged by the physician about your case presentation and your findings. In the end, you walk away, feeling devalued, disrespected, and unsure of your clinical judgment.

Nurse Practitioner:

Share with your partner how you felt during this interaction.

What would you do differently in the future?

What could you do to develop a better working relationship with the physician?

Identify what you could have done to improve communication between the physician and yourself.

Physician:

Identify possible reasons for your difficult interaction with the nurse practitioner.

Identify ways that you could have turned the interaction into a coaching moment for the nurse practitioner.

Discussion:

Discuss strategies for team building within the practice.

Identify how individual "feelings" may have gotten in the way of establishing the plan of care for the patient.

_____

_____

_____

_____

_____

_____

_____

_____

3. Evidence-Based Medicine vs. Patient-Centered Care

Pair off as patient and nurse practitioner.

The scenario is that you, the patient, have recently been discharged from the hospital after being presented with a plan of care that is totally out of reach for you to follow. You live on a fixed income, you are barely making ends meet, and you are recovering from a myocardial infarction. You cannot afford the medications that were prescribed for you during your hospitalization and you are afraid that you will further jeopardize your health by not taking the medications.

You present in the office for a follow-up visit with the nurse practitioner.

Patient:

Identify possible feelings that you may be having after this life-changing event.

How will this diagnosis change your life?

How will you make ends meet with the added costs of medications?

What are your options?

How do you ask for help?

Nurse Practitioner:

Identify communication strategies that you could employ to assist this patient.

What are your options to adjust the patient's plan of care?

How can you reassure this patient?

Identify holistic measures that you can draw from to understand the patient's situation.

Discussion:

Identify what broke down during the patient's hospitalization when the plan of care was initially developed.

Share experiences that you have had in practice that are similar to this one.

Have you been successful in communicating patient needs to other members of the healthcare team?

What has worked? And what has not worked?

_____

_____

_____

_____

_____

_____

_____

_____

4. Evidence-Based Medicine vs. Patient-Centered Care

The scenario is that you, the nurse practitioner, are assessing a patient in follow-up to determine if his chronic pain has improved. Mr. Smith started physical therapy and a regimen of pain medication 6 weeks ago. Because narcotic medications had been prescribed, a controlled substance contract was established with this patient. The patient is requesting additional pain medication because of poor pain control. However, the random urine toxicology screening performed today did not detect a trace of medication in his system. You suspect that the patient may be diverting the drugs that were prescribed.

Nurse Practitioner:

How will you approach your concerns with this patient?

What information do you have to back up your assessment?

Did you adequately explore the possible options for the negative urine toxicology screening? If not, why not?

Describe the aspects of this situation that are most disturbing for you.

JOURNALING EXERCISES

1. Interdisciplinary and Peer Communication

Describe a situation where communication broke down between you and another nurse.

What was most challenging?

How did you handle the situation?

What did you learn from this interaction?

How would you approach a similar situation?

_____

_____

_____

_____

_____

_____

_____

2. Interdisciplinary and Peer Communication

Describe a situation where you did not agree with an order that a physician has prescribed for a patient.

How did you approach the situation?

Were you successful in communicating your concern?

Did the physician collaborate with you?

Was there a positive patient outcome?

What did you learn from the scenario?

What would you do differently in the future?

_____

_____

_____

_____

_____

_____

_____

_____

3. Evidence-Based Care vs Patient-Centered Care

Describe the benefits of evidence-based care.

What works?

What are the limitations?

Describe patient-centered care.

What works?

What are the limitations?

Why is it important to blend the two models?

Share an experience where you feel that a patient has benefited from this combined approach to care.

_____

_____

_____

_____

_____

_____

_____

_____

4. Evidence-Based Care vs Patient-Centered Care

Describe a clinical situation where you questioned whether the patient was being honest with you.

What were your reactions?

Did your feelings of patient deception affect your ability to effectively communicate with the patient?

Describe how you felt during the interaction.

What would you do differently in a similar situation in the future?

Describe strategies that could be used to build trust between the patient and the provider.

REFERENCES

American Association of Colleges of Nursing. (2006). *The essentials of doctoral education for advanced nursing practice.* Washington, DC: AACN.

American College of Physicians. (2009). *Nurse practitioners in primary care.* Philadelphia: Author; Policy Monograph.

American Nurses Association. (2008). *Letter to Craig Anderson,* Chair, AMA Reference Committee B, Legislation, June 11,2008 by Rebecca Patton (President, ANA) & Linda J. Stierle, (CEO, ANA).

American Nurses Association. (2004). *Nursing: Scope and standards of practice.* Washington, DC: ANA.

APRN Joint Dialogue Group Report. (2008). Consensus model for APRN regulation: Licensure, accreditation, certification & education. National Council of State Boards of Nursing APRN Advisory Committee.

Baltimore, J. (2006). Nurse collegiality: Fact or fiction. *Nursing Management, 37*(5), 28–36.

Broome, M. E. (2005). Constructive debate and dialogue in nursing. *Nursing Outlook, 53*(4), 167–168.

Carlson, L. H. (2003). The clinical doctorate—Asset or albatross? *Journal of Pediatric Health Care, 17*(4), 216–218.

Center for American Nurses. (2007). *Lateral violence and bullying in the workplace.* Silver Spring, MD: Author.

Chase, S. K., & Pruitt, R. H. (2006). The practice doctorate: Innovation or disruption? *The Journal of Nursing Education, 45*(5), 155–161.

Clement, D. G. (2005). Impact of the clinical doctorate from an allied health perspective. *AANA Journal, 73*(1), 24–28.

Cox, K. (2001). The effects of unit morale and interpersonal relations on conflict in the nursing unit. *Journal of Advanced Nursing, 35*(1), 17–25.

Davies, B., & Hughes, A. (1995). Clarification of advanced nursing practice: Characteristics and competencies. *Clinical Nurse Specialist, 9*(3), 156–160, 166.

Dawood, M. (2005). Patient centered care: Lessons from the medical profession. *Emergency Nurse, 13*(1), 22–27.

Department of Health, Education, and Welfare Secretary's Committee to Study Extended Roles for Nurses. (1972). Extending the scope of nursing practice: A report of the secretary's committee to study extended roles for nurses. *Journal of the American Medical Association, 220*(9), 1231–1236.

Dracup, K., & Bryan-Brown, C. (2005). Doctor of nursing practice—MRI or total body scan? *American Journal of Critical Care, 14*, 278–281.

Duffy, E. (1995). Horizontal violence: A conundrum for nursing. *Journal of the Royal College of Nursing, 2*(2), 5–17.

Farrell, G. (2001). From tall poppies to squashed weeds: Why don't nurses pull together more? *Journal of Advanced Nursing, 35*(1), 26–33.

Fitzgerald, D., Mikanowicz, C., & Leslie, M. (2008). *Therapeutic communication in nursing.* Clifton Park, NY: Delmar Cengage Learning.

Freire, P. (1972). *Pedagogy of the oppressed.* England: Penguin Education.

Fulton, J. S., & Lyon, B. L. (2005). The need for some sense making: Doctor of nursing practice. *Online Journal of Issues in Nursing, 10*(3), 4.

Fried, B., Topping, S., & Rundall, T. G. (2000). Groups and teams in health services organizations. In S. M. Shortell, & A. D. Kaluzny (Eds.), *Health care management. Organization design and behavior* (4th ed). Albany, NY: Delmar.

Institute of Medicine. (2001). *Crossing the quality chasm: A new health system for the 21st century/committee on quality health care in America.* Washington, DC: Author.

International Council of Nurses. (2004). *Guidelines on coping with violence in the workplace.* Geneva, Switzerland: ICN.

The Joint Commission. (2007). Leadership chapter. Accessed May 29, 2009, from http://www.jointcommission.org/AccreditationPrograms/Hospitals/Standards/hap_prepub_stds.htm

Julia, M. C., & Thompson, A. (1994). Essential elements of interprofessional teamwork task and maintenance functions. In R. M. Casto, & M. C. Julia (Eds.), *Interprofessional care and collaborative practice.* Pacific Grove, CA: Brooks/Cole Publishing Co.

Meleis, A. I., & Dracup, K. (2005). The case against the DNP: History, timing, substance, and marginalization. *Online Journal of Issues in Nursing, 10*(3), 3.

Nelson, E., Batalden, P., & Godfrey, M. (2007). *Quality by design: A clinical microsystems approach.* San Francisco: Jossey-Bass.

Roberts, S. J. (1983). Oppressed group behavior: Implications for nursing. *Advances in Nursing Science, 5*(4), 21–30.

Sackett, D. L., Rosenberg, W. M., Gray, J. A., Haynes, R. B., & Richardson, W. S. (1996). Evidence-based medicine: What it is and what it isn't. *British Medical Journal, 312*(7023), 71–72.

Shermont, H., Mahoney, J., Krepcio, D., Baccari, S., Powers, D., & Yusha, A. (2008). Meeting of the minds: Ten-minute "huddles" of nurses and opportunity to assess unit workflow and optimize patient care. *Nursing Management, 39*(8), 38–44.

Valentine, P. (1995). Management of conflict: Do nurse/women handle it differently? *Journal of Advanced Nursing, 22*(1), 142–149.

Wilkie, W. (1996). Understanding the behavior of victimized people. In P. McCarthy, M. Sheehan, & W. Wilkie (Eds.), *Bullying, from backyard to boardroom.* Australia: Millennium Books.

CHAPTER 9

Specific Issues Related to Advanced Practice Roles

Elcha Shain Buckman

The one who count are those persons who - though they may be of little renown respond to and are responsible for the continuation of the living spirit.

—*Martin Buber*

Advanced practice nurses have the advanced academic and board certification credentials that enable them to perform fully the activities and functions of accountable, responsible, independent clinicians. Unmistakable because of the title, the purpose of this chapter is to identify the issues specifically relevant to the role of advanced practice nurses. Introduced first will be a few particular theorists whose knowledge has provided the stimuli for the tremendous growth in advanced practice nursing and in, what I term, "the field of applied advanced nursing practice." As I believe, with improbable bias, there are no drawbacks to advanced nursing practice, our focus will be totally on the advantages our credentials allow us: how we can integrate them into our practices; places we can go with them, things we can do, and ventures we can undertake that otherwise would be closed to us; and, with the aid of some of my models, what we can accomplish. Some thoughtful exercises will illustrate practical application of concept to practice.

THEORIES FOR KNOWLEDGE-BASED PRACTICE

The only person who is educated is the one who has learned how to learn and change.

—Carl Ransom Rogers

Advanced practice nursing is a relatively new level of clinical practice, coming securely into view in the mid-1970s when The National Institute of Mental Health (NIMH) offered full grants with stipends for nurses with bachelor degrees to return to specific universities for master's degrees in community psychiatric–mental health nursing. This degree would prepare them as primary psychotherapists in community and hospital settings and, then, with further experience, private practice settings. The 1980s saw expanding advanced nursing practice master's degree and nurse practitioner programs. This author did not coin the term "field of applied advanced practice nursing" until recently, after 32 years in independent private practice as a psychotherapist, university professor, and international consultant and speaker.

The 20th century saw the field of psychiatry experience two major growth periods, from the 1920s through the end of the 1940s, and again beginning in the late 1960s and continuing through today. This second spurt laid a firm foundation for advanced nursing practice which began with psychiatric nursing. Psychiatrists, psychologists, and psychiatric nurses have been the principal contributors to the practices of caring and communication with the most theoretically prominent areas being reflective practice (Buber, 1970; Buckman, 1994; Rogers, 1961; Sullivan, 1953); provider–patient relationship (Orlando, 1961; Peplau, 1952); and novice to expert (Benner, 1984; Benner, Tanner, & Chelsa, 1996). Theorists in other fields who have contributed to human caring and communication include systems theory (Bertalanffy, 1968; Selye, 1950); process consultation (Schein, 1988, 1998); and strategic intervention (Buckman, 1996).

We cannot avoid using power, cannot escape the compulsion to afflict the world, so let us, cautious in diction and mighty in contradiction, love powerfully.

—Martin Buber

Reflective Practice

Harry Stack Sullivan (1953), digressing greatly from Sigmund Freud's abstract conceptions of the unconscious mind, based his work in psychoanalysis on direct and verifiable observations. Sullivan was known to sometimes sit next to his patient so the two of them together could focus on the problem, as if it were independent of the patient, sitting in a chair opposite them. Understanding the individual as a member of a network of relationships in which he or she was enmeshed, he developed a theory of psychiatry based on interpersonal relationships where cultural and developmental forces, forming patterns of interactions with others, were largely responsible for mental illnesses. With

Sullivan's belief that one must pay detailed attention to the nuances of the *interactional*, not *intrapsychic* life of a patient, he established the theory of interpersonal psychoanalysis.

Martin Buber, Jewish theologian and philosopher, wrote *I and Thou* (1970), which has had a wide impact on people of all faiths. Living in a devoutly orthodox community, where there were constant encounters with neighbors and the world, the human "I" and the divine "Thou" formed the basis for Buber's *philosophy of dialogue* in interpersonal relationships. This dialogue can occur between man and man, man and God, and man and himself (this he termed *monologue*). Buber believed the I–Thou relationship is a dialogue with mutuality, openness, directness, and human sympathy, forming the basis of all human values. His is the first time that the focus of communication was on allowing oneself to "experience" the deepest of feelings and expressing them while actively involved in a dyadic relationship. "The major problem within our human community for the remainder of this century and into the next would be communication from polarized positions. Polarized communication can be summarized as the inability to believe or seriously consider one's own view as wrong and the other's opinion as truth" (Arnett, 1986, p. 15). According to Arnett (1986, p. vii), Buber's lifelong concern with community and the implications of dialogic communication within the context of community was at the heart of Buber's life and work.

Carl Rogers established the client-centered approach to psychotherapy in response to his observations and perceptions that the client knows what hurts, what problems are crucial, what experiences have been deeply buried, and what direction to go in. He began to rely on the client for direction in the therapeutic process (Rogers, 1951). To be effective, Rogers believed psychotherapists must be authentic and empathetic in their understanding of the patient and form a partnership around the work of therapy. His belief in his patients was so strong that he renamed patient as *client*, giving birth to his theory of client-centered, nondirective psychotherapy (Rogers, 1951). Rogers believed that the client should have as much impact on the direction of their therapy as does the psychotherapist. This approach allows the client and clinician to develop a trusting, working partnership, enabling self-acceptance. As the client begins to feel positive and accepting toward the self, defenses lower and the client becomes more open, feeling freer to grow and change in their desired path. Though best known for his client-centered approach, Rogers, with colleagues Abraham Maslow and Rollo May, established the humanistic school of psychology as reaction against the dispassionate practicing of behaviorism and psychoanalysis. Humanistic psychotherapy emphasizes the importance of self as the holding center of values, intentions, and meaning in the client's life.

Elcha Shain Buckman formed the basis for her theory that "humor is a communication facilitator" of any human emotion while growing up in a humorous

Jewish family. In her psychiatric nursing education she was fortunate to be exposed to many schools of thought and practice of psychotherapy. Blending her observations with close scrutiny of the results of her interpersonal, interactive, reflective psychotherapy practice with her clients, and detailed academic and qualitative research, Buckman (1994) began recognizing humor as reflective practice in 1964, long before developing her theoretical and practice principles that humor is a defense mechanism of the highest order, a communication facilitator of all feeling, a juxtaposition of two conflicting feelings, paradoxical, interpretive in nature, a social connector, incongruous, a brief respite from psychic pain, a sparer of psychic energy, and fun. Freud (1960) called humor our most elaborate defense mechanism and Vaillant (1971) stated it was the highest level of defense mechanism. Humor is an economic, intrapsychic process directed at simultaneously communicating and defending painful feelings that cannot be expressed seriously, momentarily sparing the client their painful feelings. Ever the observer of human reaction, Buckman cautions that humor can be hurtful but, when used carefully and selectively and then followed up with serious exploration of the underlying painful feelings, brings the client and clinician closer to each other and to the resolution of entrenched, critically painful issues.

Provider–Patient Relationship

Hildegard Peplau (1952), one of the pioneering nursing theorists, provided nursing with a meaningful method of self-directed practice at a time when nurses stood up when a physician walked in the room. Peplau's emphasis on the nurse–patient relationship as the foundation of nursing practice was seen by many as revolutionary. She formed an interpersonal model emphasizing the need for a partnership between nurse and client—as opposed to the client passively receiving treatment and the nurse passively acting out doctors' orders—and the nurse taking an active role in patient care through observation, description, formulation, interpretation, validation, and intervention and checking with the patient for accuracy of the nurse's impressions. Her model has proved of great value to later nurse theorists and clinicians in developing more sophisticated and therapeutic nursing interventions.

Peplau identified six nursing roles that illustrate the dynamic character roles typical to clinical nursing: (1) the stranger role provides an accepting climate that builds trust; (2) the resource role answers questions, interprets clinical treatment data, gives information; (3) the teaching role gives instructions and provides training; (4) the counseling role assists understanding and integrates guidance and encouragement to make changes; (5) the surrogate role clarifies domains of dependence, interdependence, and independence and acts as a patient advocate; and (6) the active leadership role helps patients assume maximum responsibility for meeting treatment goals. Peplau's developmental stages of the nurse–patient relationship are the orientation phase, the working phase, the identification phase, the exploitation phase, and the resolution phase.

Ida Jean Orlando (1961), a caring and enjoyable theorist, who every one knew was very cool before it was cool to be cool, contributed the now historic interpersonal relationships (IPR) theory that transformed provider–patient relationships. Orlando's theory was developed in the late 1950s from observations she recorded between a nurse and patient. Despite her efforts, she was only able to categorize the records as *good* or *bad* nursing. It then dawned on her that both the formulations for good and bad nursing were contained in the records. From these observations, she formulated the nursing process by identifying the role of the nurse as finding out and meeting the patient's immediate need for help. The patient's presenting behavior may not be what it appears to be; therefore, nurses need to use their perceptions, thoughts about the perceptions, and the feeling engendered from their thoughts to explore with patients the meaning of their behavior. Orlando's theory remains one of the most effective practice theories obtainable and the use of her theory keeps the nurse's focus on the patient. The strength of the theory is that it is clear, concise, and easy to use. While providing the overall framework for nursing, the use of her theory does not exclude nurses from using other theories while caring for the patient. Orlando's major concepts provide a structural base for the advanced practice nurse to do an assessment and evaluation of the patient's needs and plan interventions to meet those needs while using her perceptions, thoughts, and feelings upon which the nurse bases her actions.

Buckman, a creative entrepreneurial and innovative qualitative researcher and advanced practice nurse, has made two significant contributions to provider–client relationship theory by drawing heavily on her independent psychotherapy and business consultation practices and can be utilized in either setting. Adding interdependent as a behavioral choice, she created and tested her model of a progressive continuum on a new Buckman Independent–Interdependent–Dependent Relationship Scale™© (BIIDRS™©), along which the client moves as their developing insight and growth from the provider–patient therapy relationship impacts the changing nature of their relationships. With interdependence as an alternative reaction choice, this theory teaches the client to have control over the decisions about their reactions to disturbances in the independent–dependent relationship balance. Buckman's second provider–patient relationship theory is based on the glass-half-empty/glass-half-full perception of relationships and functioning in work and social settings. She reconstructed the "selfish–selfless" balance most of us feel some of the time into a three-point choice scale by adding her own neologism *selfsome*, meaning the client has some for themselves and therefore some for others, so the client need not feel emotionally emptied by giving away or emotionally stuffed by storing all of their emotions. The Buckman Selfish–Selfsome–Selfish Scale™© (B3S™©) three-point emotional self-measurement scale permits the client discrete evaluation of their emotions. Both scales give clients in any setting tools to measure the degree of their guilt, angry, and sad feelings regarding how they are being treated in any given relationship or situation.

Novice to Expert

Patricia Benner and Dreyfus and Dreyfus are noted for their research with people in the field of science and for identifying a five-stage skill acquisition process of novice to expert behavior. Both agree that the expert level does not mean that development stops, because expert practitioners need to evaluate their practice and keep up-to-date with new evidence.

The Dreyfus' (1986) model of skill acquisition postulates that when individuals acquire a skill through instruction, they normally pass through these five stages: novice, competence, proficiency, expertise, and mastery. In the novice stage, a person follows rules, has no discretionary judgment, and depends on abstract principles. In the practice environment, competency develops and the novice passes through three other stages (advanced beginner, competent, and proficient); when they then arrive at expert, they rely on concrete experience because they have developed an intuitive sense and their own rules. Because the Dreyfus' work closely with Benner in hospital-based nursing practice settings, they also identified seven competencies: helping role; teaching–coaching; diagnosing and patient monitoring functions; effective management of rapidly changing situations; administering and monitoring therapeutic intervention; monitoring and assuring quality of health care practices; and organizational work–role competencies (Dreyfus & Dreyfus, 1996). The progression is thus viewed as a gradual transition from rigid adherence to rules to an intuitive mode of reasoning that relies heavily on deep tacit understanding. This is shown in individuals who use intuition in decision making and develop their own rules to formulate plans.

Benner (1984, 1996) is noted for her own expert research and excellent work in adapting the Dreyfus research model to nursing practice. Benner (1984, pp. 166–167) differs slightly from Dreyfus in the naming of the categories of the five stages from novice to expert. Benner identifies these five stages of nursing practice: novice, advanced beginner, competent, proficient, and expert. She expressed that "organizational design can facilitate the care giving process of clinical experts [and] nursing is a cultural paradox in a highly technological society which is slow to value and articulate caring practice [and] feels that the value of extreme individualism makes it difficult to perceive the brilliance of caring in expert nursing practice." More recently, Benner (2004), in an abstract of her research, noted that her studies "extend the understanding of the Dreyfus model to complex, underdetermined, and fast-paced practices. The skill of involvement and the development of moral agency are linked with the development of expertise, and change as the practitioner becomes more skillful. Nurses who had some difficulty with understanding the ends of practice and difficulty with their skills of interpersonal and problem engagement did not progress to the level of expertise. Taken together, these studies demonstrate the usefulness of the Dreyfus model for understanding the learning needs and styles of learning at different levels of skill acquisition."

Caring and Communication

Communication is a form of caring behavior. In advanced practice roles both caring and communication are expected; both are a privilege and a responsibility. With the increased responsibilities and stressors that can accompany advanced practice roles, nurse clinicians can become inflexible and time constrained, regressing into familiar behavior of busy medical practices, "I don't have time to answer that" or "Just take two aspirin and call me in the morning." This type of communication denigrates the role of advanced practice nurses and the patients we care for. Our caring communication, sensitivity, and patience remain the guardians of the health care we provide and what the patient has come to expect and deserve. By taking the time, when providing physical and emotional care, to use the communication and behavioral principles of the provider–patient relationship and reflective practice, our patients receive the care they expect and deserve, and we have moved further along the continuum of novice to expert.

ADVANTAGES OF ADVANCED PRACTICE

Work is love made visible.

—Kahlil Gibran

Incorporating Credentials Into Practice Settings

Collaboration and Collaborative Practice

Advanced practice nurses can take the credit for the now trendy collaborative practice. Inadvertently, when advanced practice acts were being designed in the late 1970s, most of our states required our collaboration (a few required on-premises or within-phone-range supervision) with a physician to be able to practice "independently." Then, it seemed like a millstone of controlling restraint. Now it's au courant. The name advanced practice says it all. We have a responsibility to our profession, ourselves, and our patients to practice collaboratively. All the research corroborates the fact that collaborative practice delivers the best and safest health care. All healthcare clinicians have a responsibility to improve communication among all providers. There is no better way to do this than through collaborative practice. There are three kinds of collaborative practice (George, 2002):

1. Collaborative Care Model focuses on patient-centered care.
2. Collaborative Seminars prepare professionals for collaborative practice.
3. Negotiated Process Approach is a practice model of interactions between a group of health professionals and a community group.

I strongly urge you to explore these options because research reports that managers say their healthcare professionals are better and safer performers, they function more efficiently, and enjoy their work more than those who have no exposure to any of these models.

Peer supervision groups (Shields et al., 1985) began in the early mid-1970s to meet the needs of the growing numbers of advanced practice psychiatric nurses. All nursing specialties would benefit from this type of collaborative peer supervision. It is a form of informal rounds, the group can be homogeneous or multidisciplinary, and everyone is treated as an equal. Peer supervision is proving to benefit patients more than customary lines of reporting. Collaborative practice and peer supervision groups are just two of the perks that come with advanced practice roles.

Third-Party Reimbursement

At first, getting paid from an insurer for services rendered feels like a meritorious reward and well-earned privilege like all the other perks that come with advanced practice. After 30 years of advanced practice, I no longer take third-party payment. For psychiatry, which is treated like a bad medical stepchild, it depends on the specialty in which you practice. If it is a group collaborative practice, with a billing department, that can remove the albatross of third-party payors. If you are in a partnership private practice and you each do the billing, the headache may be back. This can be an individual decision. Because billing is fraught with all the managed care payment problems, this is a very good time to rally around a single payor universal healthcare system for America.

Commitments

Advanced practice does not stop with the degree and certification needed for advanced practice. Benner's (1984) five-stage practice theory emphasizes moving along the continuum from novice to expert. Advanced practice clinicians, by virtue of earning their credentials, make the commitment to four areas: professional growth through practice development; meaningful continuing education through course work, conference attendance, internships, residencies, and fellowships; professional contribution and growth through research which can be evidence-based, replicative, qualitative, quantitative, clinical, and scientific; and teaching, which can encompass such things as formal class room, course development, conference and journal papers, public education and speaking, lobbying for equitable affordable health care, professional privileges, or whatever interests you.

Communication

It is a top priority responsibility of every advanced practice nurse to consistently improve all communication among all providers, support people, patients, citizens, and significant others.

Places Advanced Practice Nurses Go

Educate the Public

The public, professionals, and politicians (the three Ps) still remain un-knowledgeable about our educational and credentialing rigor, steep clinical requirements, and practice privileges, or what our APRN-BC acronym stands for (Advanced Practice Registered Nurse, Board Certified). People are not sure if we are the same as, different, and more or less than physician assistants (PA). The disbelief on people's faces when they hear we can prescribe medications, laboratory tests, procedures, and treatments and that we are capable of diagnosing and treating is astounding. We need to educate and be role models for our profession everywhere we go, every time. Words and actions together is what counts.

Competition

There is not much. We have the benefit of independent practice decision making that other healthcare professionals, other than physicians, do not have. We are powerful professionals, individually and as a group. We stand for cooperation, not competition among professionals. Even though the number of advanced practice nurses is increasing, many of whom are dual-specialty credentialed, our nursing school enrollment numbers are declining, cutting off the supply chain for advanced practice. We need to encourage healthy competition for the brightest and the best to enter schools of nursing in our universities and colleges, to transfer if they are unhappy with another chosen field; support safe, innovative fast-track programs for becoming registered nurses and advanced practice registered nurses; and continue our own advancing education and professional growth so we all can meet the future challenges of health care.

Leadership

It is well-known that the more education one has, the more prepared they are to meet and participate in the challenges of being upwardly mobile in position and compensation in the world of business. Often, leadership is confused with power brokering. Leaders are found in many positions within an organization and they rely on informed influence not power. Advanced practice roles are leadership positions and carry with it the responsibilities of stewardship and choices. In advanced practice roles we are more involved with the business aspect of our organizations, thereby having greater opportunities to encourage communication and influence change.

Privileges

Independence and Autonomy

Ask yourself if advanced practice means you practice more independently or you have an independent practice. Is it the same as being autonomous in your practice? Often the distinctions are made for us by the laws of the state nurse practice acts; sometimes it is made by the lobbying efforts of these who feel threatened by us (out of ignorance or fear); sometimes it is due to misinformation. Autonomy is a feeling as much as it is a state of being—a feeling and an action, psychological and physical. To be able to use the word independent or autonomous in relation to our practice—in honor of our achievements, as a reward for our belief in ourselves and our perseverance, a recognition that we are bright and capable—is a privilege.

Responsibility

Like independence, responsibility is a privilege. Responsibility can be easily honored or abused, either way we are held accountable. Respecting the privileges of our advanced position signals our colleagues, patients, the community, and ourselves that we are trustworthy and carry responsibility safely.

What Can Be Accomplished

Role Expansion

Accomplishing one step in a multistep series encourages us to do more. It is the nature of the beast. When I was in graduate school in 1974, one of my professors said, "Show me a nurse with a master's degree and I will show you a powerful woman"—no sexism, we were all women then. I did feel powerful. We were powerful. There is nothing wrong with feeling powerful. The problem with power is it is bestowed by someone and, if it is, then it can be taken away by someone. This was not bestowed power, it was an internal power that we brought with us that we felt. Advanced practice nurses have a responsibility to respect the power, and influence, and use them wisely.

The Business of Health Care

Every business must start with a business plan that informs their strategic plan. For clinicians, it sounds daunting. I want all of you advanced practice nurses to be thankful every day that we were educated as nurses. Ours is the only profession (other than engineering) whose education is structured entirely by systems theory. Engineering is hard core, by the numbers (literally) systems theory (Bertalanffy, 1968); while nursing is applied systems theory (Selye, 1950), adapted to physical, behavioral systems. We are taught that every patient, every person, is a part, not apart, of a greater social system and that we must treat, consider at the least, the whole system if the patient is to optimally recover. Nursing is to the business of part of health care what systems theory is to engineering. Every nurse must start with nursing process. Businesses, without giving us due diligence, adapted nursing process to business and called it strategic planning. That should make your involvement with the business side of health care less daunting.

Serial Entrepreneurs

This is a fancy way of saying that some entrepreneurial people start more than one business in their lifetime. It is a title that is reserved for entrepreneurs who have had more than two successful start-up businesses. I sometimes call them my EIHs, entrepreneurs in heat—they jump on anything that moves and when it stops moving, they jump off and jump on to the next thing that moves. That means businesses stop being exciting for them when they reach a certain growth point; they get bored and look for the next business to grow. Nurses in advanced practice roles are showing signs of serial entrepreneurship. They feel that power, that excitement of achievement, of building their practice—the "fire in the belly" to the business entrepreneur—and the advanced practice nurse looks for another degree, another specialty certification, another degree in another field, another applied advanced practice nursing role. This can be a good thing.

Ventures We Can Undertake

Applied Advanced Practice Nursing

This is about transitioning one's skills and applying them to a parallel, related, or unrelated business, industry, specialty, or field. In advanced practice roles we learn to understand systems and practice from a system approach; we apply that, be it medical or business, and we understand practice, planning organization, strategizing, legalities, technology, and the list can go on. Do you want to start a medical software company, open a healthcare consulting business, go to law school, run for senator, or be a hospitalist? We learn to become experts, pushing the advocacy envelope when it benefits our patients, crossing the boundary to save a life. Use your expertise for growth and change, apply your skills to other area. Be passionate, creative, innovative, entrepreneurial, and intrapreneurial (entrepreneurial within your organization).

THE BUCKMAN BUSINESS CONSULTING MODEL™/©

I designed my business consulting model based on my concept of applied advanced practice roles. In 1978 I opened up an independent private psychotherapy practice in Cambridge, Massachusetts, and an office in my suburban home so I could be with my children more. I did this 2 years after receiving my master's degree and becoming the 36th person to be board certified. I was also in a doctoral program and was the founder and lobbyist for Nurses United for Responsible Services (NURS), the organization that got all the privileges for advanced practice psychiatric nurse passed into law in Massachusetts. In 2 years, I had a thriving child and family therapy practice, a doctorate, and I was accepted into a 2-year organization consulting and management postdoctoral fellowship. I had the fire in the belly. My therapy clients who were family business owners asked me if I did "that conflict resolution, communication thing in business?" If I could do it in broom closets and ice cream shops, I certainly could do it for a business. I was on my way to a consulting practice. Long story short, family business consulting got me into the world of mergers and acquisitions, because many family businesses were being bought and sold in the 1980s.

It was definitely time for me to structure my consulting model. I ended up with tree models I could use, depending on the needs. It felt like nursing all over again. My three models are: (1) a diagnostic model to uncover the company problems and ills (Figure 9-1); (2) a strategic planning and implementation model that uses a SWOT analysis (strengths, weaknesses, opportunities and threats) (Figure 9-2 and Table 9-1); and (3) a contingency planning model (Figure 9-3).

Figure 9-1

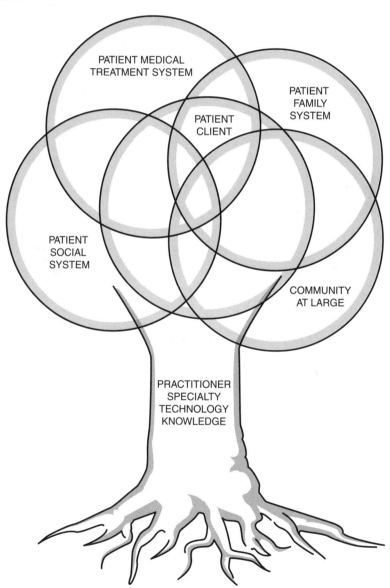

Figure 9-2

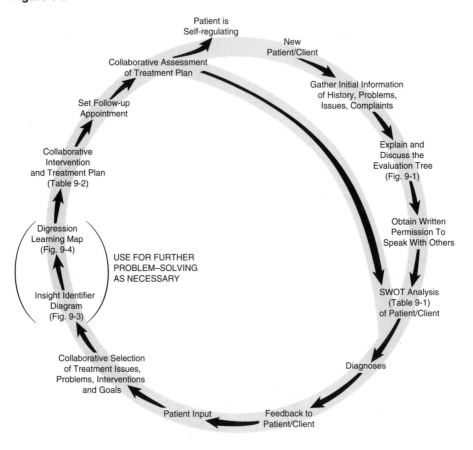

Table 9-1   SWOT Analysis

STRENGTHS (Patient/Client/Internal organization)	OPPPORTUNITIES (Patient's support system; external marketplace)
WEAKNESSES (Patient/client/organization; physical/ psychological; barriers to intervention)	THREATS (Barriers compromising change and growth; barriers to entry into marketplace)

Table 9-2   Collaborative Intervention and Treatment Plan

Intervention/Goal Statement _____

Tasks and Steps Needed to Accomplish this Goal	Person(s) Responsible for Implementing Each	Drop Dead Date (Date due to be done)	Measurement of Completion of Task/Step

Use for each intervention and goal.

Figure 9-3

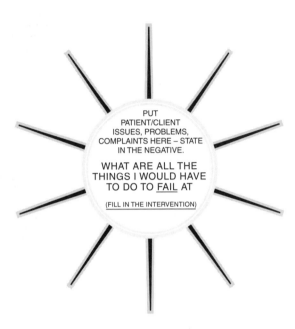

Figure 9-4

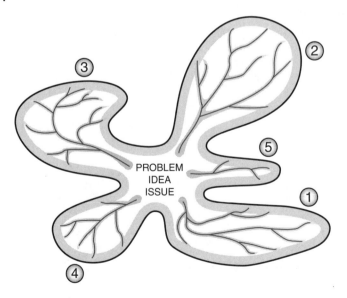

COMMUNICATION EXERCISES

1. Role Play

You are mentoring a group of five master's and thee doctoral nursing students, all with differing experience levels. You meet with them every clinical day and discuss how Dreyfus and Dreyfus' and Benner's theories of novice to expert and competencies, and Benner's concern about nursing's extreme individualism and systems theory, would affect assessment and decisions about their needs and learning goals.

Discussion:

What do they say about themselves?
Is there any difference in the way they view their levels of expertise and the way you do?
What competencies would you expect at which of the five stages?

_____

_____

_____

_____

_____

_____

_____

_____

2. Intrapreneurial

Depending on your workplace, with three other teammates create a three-goal strategic plan for one of these: a new department, new position, introducing a new product or treatment, or retrofit a building for clinic.

_____

_____

_____

_____

_____

_____

_____

_____

3. Role Play

Select a mixed group of eight colleagues plus yourself, with only one profession each represented, and make sure to include one whose specialty is psychiatry or psychology, and have two to three novices with the rest being experts. This group will consist of the person whose specialty is psychiatry or psychology—this person can be from nursing, medicine, psychology, or social work—C-level administration, nursing, medicine, pharmacy, imaging, discharge planning, rehabilitation, and a representative who is active in the community at large. Being at the expert level, and using the Buckman Business Model, you will lead a SWOT analysis to solve a clinical dilemma or organizational issue.

_____

_____

_____

_____

_____

_____

_____

4. Role Play

Your consulting company has grown and now you, your per diem consultant, and administrative assististant need help. Growth is a must to survive.

Discussion:

What strategic planning and intervention practices will you use and how will you decide?
How will you handle the following?

- What are your feelings about this crossroad?
- How many and who do you need to help you with designing the new business plan?
- What kind of consulting growth do you want?
- Company re-missioning and goals.

- What strengths and opportunities do you need?
- What will be your plan to manage the weaknesses and threats?

_____

_____

_____

_____

_____

_____

_____

_____

5. Consultation Team

Your four-member team has a suddenly strident client you have been work-ing with for 4 months. It has been a good experience for consultants and client organization. The client is a family owned handicap product manu-facturing company with one engaged son, two daughters, one son-in-law, and the founding mother is still around; there are 20 employees. Your con-sultation team has hit a snag—a series of small events have piled on top of each other to the point that every one thinks it is a riot of errors. The team considers using humor as the intervention.

Discussion:

What kind?
If so, how and why?
If not, why not? What would you do?
Do you have a contingency plan? What is it?

_____

_____

_____

_____

_____

_____

_____

_____

JOURNALING EXERCISES

Set three professional goals and how you will achieve them.

Design a strategic plan to run for a public office of your choosing.

Identify a business you would like to start-up and outline a business plan for it.

Finish the lists in the applied nursing practice section.

As a novice, identify a professional organization sponsoring a local conference, outline "Applying evidence-based research results to clinical practice" paper, and prepare a letter to the conference chairperson.

As an expert, prepare a 2-minute lobbying speech to be presented to our national House of Representatives defining why advanced practice nurses need to be included on the task force for healthcare reform.

REFERENCES

Arnett, R. C. (1986). *Communication and community: Implications of Martin Buber's dialogue.* Carbondale, IL: Southern Illinois University Press.

Benner, P. (1984). *From novice to expert: Excellence and power in clinical nursing practice.* Menlo Park, CA: Addison-Wesley.

Benner, P., Tanner, C. A., & Chesla C. A. (1996). *The relationship of theory and practice in the acquisition of skill.* New York: Springer Publishing Co.

Benner, P. (2004). Using the Dreyfus model of skill acquisition to describe and interpret skill acquisition and clinical judgment in nursing practice and education. *Bulletin of Science, Technology & Society, 24*(3), 188–199.

Buber, M. (1970). *I and thou.* (W. Kaufmann, Trans.). New York: Charles Scribner's Sons.

Buckman, E. S. (1994). *Handbook of humor: Clinical applications in psychotherapy.* Malabar, FL: Krieger.

Buckman, E. S. (1996). What's your social IQ. In J. M. Baldwin (Ed.), *What your little black book tells you* (pp. 24–43). New York: SFC Communications Corporation.

Dreyfus, H. L., & Dreyfus, S. E. (1986). *Mind over machine: The power of human intuition and expertise in the age of the computer.* Oxford: Basil Blackwell.

Dreyfus, H. L., & Dreyfus, S. E. (1996). Expertise in nursing practice: Caring, clinical judgment, and ethics. In P. Benner, C. A. Tanner, & C. A. Chesla (Eds.), *The relationship of theory and practice in the acquisition of skill* (pp. 29–40). New York: Springer.

Freud, S. (1960). *Jokes and their relation to the unconscious.* New York: W. W. Norton.

George, J. (Ed.). (2002). *Nursing theories: The base for professional practice* (5th ed.). Upper Saddle River, NJ: Prentice Hall.

Orlando, I. J. (1961). *The dynamic nurse-patient relationship, function, process and principles.* New York: G. P. Putnam.

Peplau, H. (1952). *Interpersonal relations in nursing.* New York: Springer Publishing Co.

Rogers, C. R. (1951). *Client-centered therapy.* Boston: Houghton Mifflin.

Rogers, C. (1961). *On becoming a person: A therapist's view of psychotherapy.* London: Constable.

Schein, E. J. (1988). *Process consultation revisited: Building the helping relationship* (2nd ed.). Reading, MA: Addison-Wesley.

Schein, E. J. (1998). *Process consultation: It's role in organizational development.* Reading, MA: Addison-Wesley.

Selye, H. (1950). *The physiology and pathology of exposure to stress.* Montreal, Quebec, Canada: Acta, Inc.

Shields, J., Gavrin, J., Hart-Smith, V., Kombrink, L., Kovach, J., Sheeehan, M., et al. (1985). *Peer consultation in a group context: A guide for professional nurses.* New York: Springer Publishing Co.

Sullivan, H. S. (1953). *The interpersonal theory of psychiatry.* New York: W. W. Norton.

Vaillant, G. E. (1971).Theoretical hierarchy of adaptive ego mechanisms. *Archives of General Psychiatry, 24,* 107–117.

Von Bertalanffy, L. (1968). *General systems theory.* New York: Braziller.

SUGGESTED READINGS

Eraut, M. Quoted in G. Cheetham and G. E. Chivers (2005). *Professions, competence and informal learning* (p. 162). Northampton, MA: Edward Elgar Publishing.

Frankl, V. E. (1984). *Man's search for meaning* (3rd ed.). New York: Simon & Schuster, Inc.

Fry, W. F. (1963). *Sweet madness.* Palo Alto, CA: Pacific Books.

Martin, Rod A. (2007). *The psychology of humour: An integrative approach.* London, UK: Elsevier Academic Press.

Maslow, A. (1970). *Motivation and personality* (2nd ed.). New York: Harper and Row.

Mindess, H. (1971). *Laughter and liberation.* Los Angeles: Nash.

Neuman, B., & Fawcett, J. (Eds.). (2002). *The Neuman systems model* (4th ed.). Upper Saddle River, NJ: Prentice Hall.

Oberlander, J. (2003). *Political life of Medicare.* Chicago: University of Chicago Press.

Parker, M. E. (Ed.). (2001). *Nursing theories and nursing practice.* Philadelphia: F.A. Davis Co.

Tomey, A. M., & Alligood, M. R. (Eds.). (2002). *Nursing theorists and their work* (5th ed.). St. Louis, MO: Mosby.

Ziv, A. (1984). *Personality and a sense of humor.* New York: Springer Publishing Co.

CHAPTER 10

Communication and Peer Group Supervision

Valerie A. Hart

I first experienced the value of participating in a peer group when I accepted my first position after graduate school as a Psychiatric–Mental Health Clinical Specialist at McLean Hospital in 1977. I was invited to join an ongoing group that originally consisted of former graduate students from Boston University. The group had formed in 1974 in order to address role pressure that is inherent for any group of professionals who are carving out new roles. In this case, individuals worked in a variety of settings, with the common denominator of a graduate degree and national certification in a specialty area of nursing. The group met on a weekly basis for the purpose of providing supervision in a new model—that of a peer group. Prior methods of obtaining supervision for clinical work had been working with a mentor or supervisor, usually a psychiatrist. Members of this group worked in a wide array of settings including private practice, large university medical centers, a public university, a counseling center, and a psychotherapy institute. Many members felt the isolation of being the only Psychiatric–Mental Health Clinical Specialist among a sea of other professionals. In addition to providing psychotherapy, members were educators, consultants, supervisors, and department heads. The process of conducting case reviews, as well as the exploration of role-related dilemmas, made for exciting meetings. The group knew we were in novel territory that was highly creative and we wanted to share it with a wider audience.

The new model seemed to produce something dynamic and exciting and the group was thriving. Members all knew of other peer groups that had formed and then floundered, and we began to speculate about why our group was successful. After meeting for 10 years, the group made a commitment to define and document a new model of providing peer supervision. Finding a publisher was challenging initially, because we received feedback that the work was too intellectual for nurses. Refusing to believe this, we ventured forth and, since perseverance is often the key to publication, we eventually prevailed. *Peer Consultation in a Group Context* (Shields et al., 1985) was the result. It was meant as a handbook for other professionals who might benefit from this form of professional development. Although all chapters have individual members' names assigned as lead author, the book was a group effort. After all, we were trying to make a point about collaboration and group work. We pushed the publisher to have a *group picture* on the back cover in order to drive this point home.

Since that first peer group, I have participated in two other peer groups; the composition of my next group and my current group consist of an eclectic mix of disciplines, including psychologists, social workers, and licensed counselors. Instead of the common denominator being that of advanced practice nurses, it became the role of psychotherapists.

PEER GROUPS

This chapter will outline a model of peer supervision which can provide ongoing professional development for the healthcare provider, regardless of discipline. In researching this topic I found that beyond health care, peer groups are advertised and advocated for a wide array of professionals.

Tisdall and O'Donoghue (2003) describe a facilitated peer group for New Zealand providers working in the field of family violence. While the concept of peer supervision was originally conceived by those in the psychiatric–mental health field, the power of its effectiveness has spread wide and far.

In doing an online search, I found peer groups for small business owners, personnel and project managers, massage therapists, certified public accountants, sales managers, educators, public relations specialists, chief executive officers (CEOs), consultants, school counselors, information technology professionals, corporate executives, and home remodelers, as well as the usual healthcare professionals. The *Peer Group* is a moderated peer program for the bio-pharmaceutical industry that hosts events for healthcare professionals. Its services include moderator led dinner meetings, teleconferences, Web conferences, and lunch and learn programs. A spring 2006 newsletter for clinical psychologists, *Times–Philadelphia Society of Clinical Psychologists* (PSCP), had the following ad:

> *New Peer Consultation Group: This group is a general peer consultation group open to any interested PSCP member. Meetings will take place monthly during day time hours at The Center in King of Prussia.*

The Public Relations Society of America (PRSA) launched peer groups in 2006 in order to:

provide an opportunity for practitioners to get together and share needs, ideas, vendors and professional resources, and more. The Groups are:

1. *Corporate Peer Group: for members who are corporate communicators;*
2. *Firm Peer Group: for those who are principals or staff in a public relations firm, or those who are sole practitioners, consultants, or freelancers;*
3. *Non-Profit and Government Professionals: for members working in non-profit/not-for-profit organizations: hospitals, charities, educational institutions, government agencies, trade associations and more.*

In addition, if there is interest we will launch a New Professionals Peer Group, for members who have less than eight years' experience in public relations.

About the Peer Groups

Your peers understand your challenges and issues. Like-minded, achievement-oriented individuals can help you leverage your strengths and experience. Two heads are better than one—and six, eight or ten heads are even better.

Each Peer Group will create an agenda of topics and then discuss each subject among its members or with an invited "expert." For example, the PR Firms / Sole Practitioners Peer Group might choose to explore (a) Retaining and growing clients; (b) Winning business against tough competition; (c) Vendors worth knowing (graphic designers, Web site developers, printers, computer experts, accountants, etc.); (d) Managing Time and Quality; and (e) Marketing, Positioning, Strategy, Differentiation, Program Creation.

There are no dues or fees for the Peer Groups: your only cost is your own meal at meetings and your share of the cost of an occasional guest-expert's meal.

Benefits of attending the Groups

- *Enjoy the support and encouragement of a network of successful people to move your projects, career or business forward.*
- *Bounce ideas off others and get helpful feedback before you take action—saving time, energy and money.*

- *Increase your chances of reaching your own goals, as a group of people with the same challenges help you create solutions and action steps.*
- *Benefit from better decision-making and problem solving. Find solutions from proactive, objective people who want you to succeed. Your peers will be a unique brain trust of people who have been there and done that.*

The Painting and Decorating Contractors of America (PDCA) has a peer group curriculum that promises "an avenue for continuous improvement" as a result of sharing best practices. This material is combined with coaching and a peer group. According to their Web page:

PDCA peer group costs are substantially less than other programs. Other groups charge anywhere from $8,000 to over $20,000 annually and they do not have the proven curriculum, planning software, financial analysis and performance tracking. PDCA programs have one focus—member profitability.

Joining a Peer Group is Easy

PDCA peer groups are made up of non-competing painting contractors from different geographic locations with a common thread such as size, how services are delivered, or construction specialty. A PDCA peer group is like having a board of directors for your company made up of sub-contractors just like yourself, who want your business to succeed as much as they want their own businesses to succeed.

The secrets to successful peer groups are three key components:

- *The group must be mixed and matched based upon disciplines and goals.*
- *The peer group must be managed and facilitated.*
- *Each peer group participant must be genuinely interested in sharing information about best practices, listening to other members about their challenges, and committing full attention to the group process.*

The Collaborative Peer Supervision Group Project, based in Columbus, Ohio, is a model partially based on our original model and an initiative to improve communication between pediatricians and child psychiatrists at the National Center for Infants, Toddlers and Families, known as Zero To Three (Thomasgard, Warfield, & Williams, 2004).

The Goldhill Group offers peer groups for CEOs. Their Web page explains:

> *The peer advisory board experience has proven to be one of the best forums for success. It offers entrepreneurs a unique opportunity to explore issues and learn in a non-competitive environment, with a group of fellow business leaders who support each other in improving their lives, businesses and organizational effectiveness.*

Program Features:

> *Meet once per month as group for 5–6 hours (7:30am–1pm)*
> *Meet once/month in your office for a private session (90–120 min.)*
> *Groups consist of 8–16 members from various industries and backgrounds*
> *Expert guest speakers who share the latest strategies and perspectives at periodic events*
> *Introductions to resources like expert consultants, business specialists, etc.*
> *Affordably priced at $750 per month*
> *Meeting location rotates; most meetings held in San Fernando Valley.*

Darrell Zahorsky (a small business expert, author, and consultant) writes a blog, facilitates a forum on the Web, and writes a small business newsletter. He extols the value of a peer advisory group composed of small business owners from diverse industries who get together monthly in order to "solve problems, share best practices, and offer each other peer support." There are qualifications for admission to a group, and the cost varies from $700 to $10,000 a year. Examples include:

Chief Executive Officers Club: members must have 2 million dollars in annual sales and membership is invitation-only.

Young Entrepreneurs' Organization: must be under 40 years old and have annual gross sales exceeding $1 million and is invitation-only.

TEC International: is in 14 countries with two peer groups. One for CEOs of companies of $5 million and up, and the other for emerging entrepreneurs with $1 million to $5 billion in revenue. Membership dues are $10,000 and it is invitation-only.

Inner Circle: for companies with revenue between $500,000 and $50 million, membership fee is between $5600 and $7500.

Women Presidents' Organization: for successful women business owners, membership is $1250 annually.

Joe Mancuso, President of CEO Club, Inc., summarizes the benefits of peer groups: "it is okay to be independent but there is no reason to be alone. We like to say it is okay to make money if you are having fun."

The Edward Lowe Foundation holds Roundtable peer group called PeerSpectives:

Recognized nationwide as an expert on peer learning, we understand the value of interacting with and learning from colleagues who often face similar leadership and business problems. That's why we developed and license the PeerSpectives Roundtable System, an innovative peer-to-peer learning tool using a proven format that focuses on sharing experiences instead of giving advice.

We know the system works, because we've seen the results first-hand in tables running in Wisconsin, Michigan, Indiana, Ohio and Florida. PeerSpectives is also a part of nearly every leadership retreat offered at Big Rock Valley. Its power to initiate discussions and ultimate solutions continues to amaze us as we watch one person after the other find those "ah ha" moments using the process. To see the process at work, view the video.

PeerSpectives Roundtables are typically comprised of 10 to 12 individuals from non-competing companies. The system is licensed by nonprofit membership and economic development groups, educational institutions or for-profit entities seeking a new resource to offer members, alumni, clients and customers.

Facilitators are key to each table's success. That's why these individuals are trained in the PeerSpectives System by the foundation. Each license covers training for one facilitator, and three training sessions are offered throughout the country each year.

The site allows users to find other CEO's in their state in order to form a peer group.

It is easy to see that peer groups come in a variety of shapes and sizes. Some are facilitated or led, and others are not. Some are mixed discipline and others are more homogenous. Regardless of composition, peer participation has become big business!

Reasons to Join a Peer Group

The concept of peer groups, for the purpose of supervision, was first conceptualized in the psychiatric–mental health field.

The cited values of peer groups are often similar—those of decreasing isolation, sharing ideas, receiving support, and building professional network. Other reasons to consider a peer group include opportunities to receive feedback on professional or clinical issues and building a professional support network. Kombrink (1985) also cites job stress, an interest in studying and resolving complex clinical encounters, quality assurance, and an opportunity to blend personal and professional goals as motivation to join a group. In most academic health-related programs, students are introduced to the notion of lifelong learning due to the rapidly shifting nature of health care. Professional development never really concludes and the same can be said about the potential for growth as a peer group member. There is a mandate to stay current in regard to clinical interventions and having a cadre of colleagues who are available for consultation is a cost-effective way to assure that this can occur. Borders (1991) identifies skill development, instructive feedback, and self-monitoring among reasons to join a peer group. Benshoff (1994) summarized research that found that peer group participation decreased dependency on expert supervisors and increased self-confidence and self-direction as beneficial outcomes. Increasing multicultural competence has also been identified as a potential outcome (Lassiter, Napolitano, Culbreth, & Ng, 2008). In one study based at a health center, findings suggested that exploring workplace conflict, professional boundaries, and emotional distress was effectively accomplished in a peer group emotional pain (Phelan, Barlow, & Iverson, 2006). Counselman and Weber (2004) cite interpersonal learning from peers, networking, support, and reducing professional isolation as further benefits of peer supervision groups.

Self-regulation, an essential component for professional practice, is linked to peer review for advanced practice registered nurses where a Peer Review Committee was formed (Kenny, Baker, Lanzon, Stevens, & Yancy, 2008). Briggs, Heath, and Kelly (2005) relate peer review to professionalism and clinical competency for advanced practice nurses.

The advanced practice nurse Peer Review Committee and the review process were developed to provide peer input and communication to all credentialed advanced practice nurses in incidents regarding appropriateness of care and scope of practice.

An additional reason to join a peer group is the ability to count it as professional activities for purposes of certification and advancement on one's resume, as it documents a commitment to professional development and lifelong learning.

Small Group Theory

In the beginning stage of group development, members establish norms for the group and deal with boundary issues. Confidentiality, discussions about friendly or respectful dialogue, and the task of the group are the typical topics of discussion. Group members will also naturally gravitate to either an intellectual or more emotional subgroup, depending on their personality. These two subgroups must make peace with one another in order for the group to survive. The group as a whole grapples with the issue of how trustworthy other members are and the group in general. Once these issues are determined the group gets down to the business at hand, regardless of what type of group it might be. This second stage is the working stage of the group. Meetings become productive as the group accomplishes the tasks that brought members into the group. In the case of peer consultation the group is leaderless and, because of this fact, some of the usual struggle with the identified leaders is avoided. Instead of a mini-revolt, which is entirely predictable according to small group theory, all of the members of the group see themselves as leaders. Because roles of host, consultee, and consultant shift from meeting to meeting, and within the same meeting, there is a shared responsibility for the functioning and success of the meetings and for the group. Hunt and Issacharoff (1975) document this dynamic in a peer group of psychotherapists. Their hypothesis is that, by being leaderless, group members develop a dependency on one another and toward the group.

Peer Consultation and Peer Supervision

Most professionals are familiar with the concept of supervision, as it is a typical configuration found in any workplace. Clinical supervision is simply focused on clinical issues, but is a process of two individual working together, one having more status, experience, or power. In graduate school, clinical supervision is done between student and professor. In a clinic, this process occurs between a supervisor and employee. Supervisors may or may not be mentors, since mentors are typically chosen by the mentee and not assigned. The purpose of having a clinical supervisor is to receive information, guidance, and professional growth. The results of supervision may or may not be tied to monetary incentives, such as annual evaluations. In the academic setting the results are tied to a certain grade in a course, either numerical grades or pass/fail. The common denominator is that there is a more experienced person evaluating a less experienced person. Supervision can be from another individual in the same discipline, or in another discipline, who possesses knowledge and experience that the supervisee requires.

Consultation is similar to supervision in that one person seeks the assistance of another who is seen as knowledgeable or expert in a certain area. The vital difference is in the lack of a power differential inherent in this process. In fact, the consultee may be viewed as being the consumer and, in the process of consultation, is free to either utilize or disregard the recommendations of the consultant. There is a basic tenet that all consultants must grapple with. It is that their viewpoint can be respectfully ignored, even if understood by the client or the person paying for the service. In the case of peer group consultation the real power to act rests with the consultee, not the consultant.

PEER GROUP CONSULTATION MODEL

The concept of a peer involves another individual with similar educational preparation and role responsibility. It does not have to mean in the same discipline. It does mean that no conflicts of interest exist or power relationships between peers. While one could presumably be a supervisor in another department they could not be supervising someone and consider them a peer for the purposes of this model. During the process of group consultation there is one consultee and the other members of the group are in the role of consultants.

Group Size and Composition

Small group theory sets the optimal size of a functioning small group at between seven to nine members. As noted previously, the members will be peers and have common role functions. When recruiting in the formation stage of the group, it is wise to begin with a larger number (10–12) in order to account for possible early attrition in the group. In groups of this size the principle of "individual challenge in the least-sized group" means that group size needs to be such that all members feel essential to the work of the group as well as rewarded for participation (Kovach, 1985). It is important for members in the group to be able to present to the group when needed. Limiting the size of the group also allows for frequent opportunities to be the consultee. Because this model is a leaderless group, the predictable dynamics that occur with the presence of a designated leader are avoided. In essence, all of the members are the leader and therefore assume responsibility for the success of the group and its functioning.

The members may be drawn from a common pool, such as a graduate school class or a work setting. It may be a more interesting group to be diverse in regard to both work sites as well as roles. There are advantages and disadvantages for a group composed of members from the same discipline. For example, having a peer group of individuals who have a doctoral in nursing practice (DNP), with various clinical specialties represented, would be useful as members carve out new roles in a variety of settings. They would share the common educational background and potential for leadership in nursing. Another group might have only those who have a DNP in pediatrics. This group would have the opportunity to not only consult with one another about role issues but clinical cases as well. Issues of prescribing to a very specific population could easily be managed. The disadvantage is that the group would lose the perspective of another discipline and another view of both organizational as well as clinical problems.

Another peer group could be composed of professionals who represent different disciplines but who work in a particular setting. For example, professionals who work in hospice, including nursing, social work, psychology, gerontology, pastoral counseling, etc., would have the advantage of members understanding at a deep level the clinical dilemmas. While there may be less opportunity to explore professional role strain and development, the breadth of clinical perspectives would be advantageous. In terms of recruitment for new group members, the model of sponsorship is useful. In this model a potential new member is recommended by a current member who is familiar with the person's professional expertise and experience and personal characteristics. Allowing members to review a potential member's resume or curriculum vitae is helpful in introducing them to the group. Adding new members to an existing group can be tricky, and it is wise to take time with this decision, as the addition of a disruptive member can have a destructive effect on the group. The sponsor can be responsible for orienting the new member to the format used for presenting in the group as well as obligations related to attendance or absences.

Skills Required for Peer Group Members

For the majority of time, the group members will function in the role of consultants; therefore, the skills of being a consultant are critical. Skills of being a consultee are also important (Table 10-1). For all members of the group, skills include an ability to make a long-term commitment to the group, make attendance a priority, and to share in the responsibility for the functioning of the group.

Housekeeping Decisions

Where to meet is one of the first decisions a group will need to consider. A system of rotation among group member's offices or a conference room at the workplace of members is a typical choice. This can facilitate the role of host for each meeting. The role of host is that of calling the meeting to a beginning, and keeping track of the time during the meeting. The question of providing light refreshments, provided by the host, can be another task that can set the tone of welcoming others to a setting and "breaking bread" together can create a special bond.

The management of social conversations and sharing personal issues is best accomplished by providing a time-limited social component to the meeting. This can be scheduled for one-half hour before the official meeting begins and be voluntary, for those who choose to come early and participate. Putting clear

Table 10-1   Skills of Consultant and Consultee

Consultant	Consultee
Ability to decide if the question that the consultee is asking is congruent with the presentation, or essential facts are being overlooked	Ability to state a crisp question for the consultants
Ability to ask questions pertaining to the question at hand in a respectful and nonjudgmental manner	Ability to structure the flow of the consultation
Ability to give suggestions in a productive way	Self-awareness of strengths and areas of personal vulnerability, specifically when functioning in a group
Ability to let go of your ideas if the consultee is not receptive to your suggestions	Ability to receive specific questioning regarding your thinking about issues
Ability to listen to the consultee's statement of the problem and the presentation that follows	Ability to tolerate different views regarding the problem as well as potential solutions

boundaries around the issue of socializing is a good way to avoid the pitfall of the peer group morphing into just a social gathering or worse, a forum for complaining about work or patients.

Being on time is an important norm for the group. If not addressed or taken lightly, members may grow to resent arriving on time and then having to wait until tardy members are present. Ending on time is just as important as starting on time. Members often have multiple demands on time and adhering to a set agreement is a way to respect this reality.

A typical group of seven to nine members will function effectively if the meeting time is 1.5 to 2 hours in length. This will allow for three to four members to present during the meeting. The meeting should start by asking who *needs* to present, and who would *like* to present. This will help the host to know how much time each consultation can have during the meeting. Often, members will communicate that they would like to present an issue or case if there is time and, if not, it can wait for the next meeting. There are times that it feels quite urgent to present, since a clinical intervention needs to be decided quickly and waiting is not an option. This type of triage of the group is efficiently done by going around the group and having each member state their needs at the beginning of the group. Negotiating time is another skill that all group members will need to cultivate. It is obviously important to address the needs of members who have an urgent request to present.

What is discussed in group needs to remain private and confidential. There needs to be agreement about not talking about the group outside of the meetings if members choose to socialize outside of meetings. The only way to assure a sense of safety is to be absolutely firm about this requirement for confidentiality.

Format of Presenting: Consultee

Gavrin (1985) identifies the inner feelings of presenting which include being the center of attention, apprehension at publicizing inner feelings, and problems in a group. She also reminds us that the sense of accomplishment, self-esteem, productivity, and validation of one's work are also the rewards of presenting to the group. The key to presenting to the group is in shaping the presentation and thinking carefully about what question you are really asking to be addressed. This requires the courage to self-disclose and admit when you are confused or having negative reactions to a patient or colleagues related to the question. Formulating the question is the most important component that the consultee needs to consider. Once this is communicated to the group, the real consultation is off and running. It is recommended that consultants do not interrupt the consultee for a period of time. Once the initial material is presented, group members can be free to ask for more information in order to clarify or put the issues into the proper context. Interrupting the consultee too early can feel challenging and make them lose focus of the question. Consultants can jot down questions to be asked so that they do not forget to do so. The process of the consultation will always revert back to the question asked by the consultee, and that is why it is the critical component. Merely launching into a description of a case or clinical situation without a focus will make the proceeds murky and lead to potential miscommunication and misunderstanding. Being able to focus on the question, in a laser-like fashion, will also help to limit the time for the consultation, allowing others to have the opportunity to present during the meeting. Since the host will be the taskmaster, in charge of keeping the time, the other members can be free to not watch the clock and let the process evolve. If the consultee does not begin with a question, it is suggested that a group member specifically ask, "What is your question?" Once the question is clear then the context of the case or situation needs to be described to the group.

While the consultee may be intimately familiar with these aspects the group members will not have this information, and will need it in order to provide constructive consultation. In structuring the order of the presentation, Gavrin (1985) suggests:

Identify the type of problem
Describe background information
Communicate your concerns
Provide a history of the problem
Share personal experiences that are related to the problem
Open up the floor for group discussion

The Consultative Process

The dynamics of a consultation follow an evolutionary model consisting of several phases (Zagata, 1985). These include:

Description, or the question
The question behind the question
The evolving hypothesis
Summary and evaluation

The first phase is self-explanatory and involves a thorough description of the issue, statement of the question, and background information. During this phase consultants listen and observe both verbal and nonverbal cues of the consultee. After the initial statements, consultants ask questions in order to clarify either the question or the context of the issue.

The question behind the question involves the implied messages in the presentation. If consultants are picking up something other than the stated question, they can attempt to renegotiate the initial question, sometimes broadening and sometimes narrowing the scope of the question. However, it is the consultee who decides what is to be addressed by the group.

During the evolving hypothesis phase various group members build, often without conscious effort, a working hypothesis of what the issues are, which lead to potential solutions of the issues. Often the perspective of one group member will trigger thoughts in another member, who will add their thoughts to the working hypothesis, thus furthering its development. This is the most dynamic portion of the consultation. It is usually energetic and lively, and members may vie for the floor wishing to jump in and add their thoughts. It is important for one or two members to not hog the floor, and for all to be allowed to contribute who wish to do so. It is not required for all members to weigh in on the topic, but monopolizing the conversation needs to be avoided.

During the summary and evaluation phase a review of the potential solutions derived from the group discussion is stated. Various strategies can be weighed and evaluated for merit in terms of addressing the original question as stated by the consultee. Complete consensus does not always occur, as members may differ in their ideas of how to proceed. This is always done with the respect of the other in mind, and knowledge that the consultee is free to choose either solution, or none at all. Again, the heart of consultation is the freedom of the consultee to make the final choice. It is also not necessary for the consultee to state what they intend to do about the issue on the spot. The consultee may need time to make the decision, and can bring an end to the consultation by simply thanking the group for the discussion and the time. The meeting then moves on to the next consultee and consultation.

Organizing the Peer Group Meeting

After providing time for socialization, the meeting should be called to order by the host peer. Each group member checks in and identifies if they have any cases or issues they would like to present. After all the members have been heard from, the host asks the identified members to prioritize their request to present and an overall schedule for the meeting is developed, including the order of presentations as well as the time that is available.

The meeting then consists of the process of consultees presenting and consultants responding. Before members convene there is a verification of the host for the next meeting.

Summary of typical meeting:

Socialization
Checking in
Prioritizing presentations
Consultations
Plans for next meeting verified

Confrontation and Competition

Confrontation is usually a term that makes palms sweat, but an issue that needs to be approached with maturity and courage. Within the course of any group there will be issues that need to be raised that would seem to make waves of some sort. In peer consultation, the situation often relates the experience of the consultee being resistant to hearing what the group is saying. This can be seen when, after the group discusses a complex issue for a length of time, the consultee changes the subject, rationalizes, or is in denial of the facts (Sheehan, 1985). At this juncture the group has the option of simply dropping the matter or confronting it in the group. If the issue is not significant to the consultation, can be reworked at a future time, or if confrontation would be damaging to either the consultee or to the group, the former option is advised. While confrontation causes anxiety, it also can afford both the individual and the group opportunities for growth that would not otherwise occur.

An important component of any effective group is the issue of feeling safe in the group. Only if members feel safe will they be willing to self-disclose and take risks. It is within this safe environment that confrontation can be of value. Sheehan (1985) gives an example of the use of confrontation in a peer group. A consultee was insisting that she needed to give up her position as a faculty member as a result of a disagreement regarding curriculum issues. The group confronted the member with the fact that she had a history of leaving positions after struggling with authority figures at work. This initially angered the consultee and she shared thoughts of leaving the group. This led to a discussion by group members of times in their professional lives when they felt helpless and trapped. Tensions calmed and members discussed how each expressed anger. Warmth and laughter soon replaced the tension and anger, and the group advanced to a new level of trust and sharing as a result of facing a sensitive issue. Remembering the mandate for confidentiality, episodes of confrontation are never discussed outside of the group.

Competition, another sensitive topic, is also essential to navigate if the group is to survive. It is not possible to avoid competitive feelings or even acting out of competitive urges that are unconscious. It is not the appearance of competition that poses the problem, it is the avoidance of the issue or the failure to manage these situations (Hart-Smith, 1985). While competition can conjure up notions of energy, excitement, and productivity, the word also can be seen as aggression, as in winning and losing. Actually the Latin root *competere* means "to seek together," which is the opposite of squaring off in order to defeat the other. The research of early social scientists regarding cooperation and competition find that individual productivity and learning do not suffer in groups that are competitive. While this may be true in a peer group, the aim is to develop an overall cooperative atmosphere while finding a way to handle competitive stirrings.

Each group member will arrive with a specific relationship to the concept of competition. The majority of this framework is forged in the family of origin. Group members can reflect on how competition was managed in their family. Was it encouraged or discouraged? Were members rewarded or shamed in regard to competing? Was this related to winning or losing? What was the overall message regarding competing with others in sports, board games, in attracting a sexual partner? In one's adult personal life is competition enjoyed or avoided? What is the individual's history of competitive situations in the workplace? How would members describe themselves in terms of competition? This knowledge helps form who we are, our personality, and how we relate to competitive situations.

An obvious time when competition can arise during a consultation is after the consultee completes their presentation of the problem and awaits discussion by group members. Competitive behavior can manifest itself in terms of the best hypothesis of what is occurring, or the best idea or solution to the problem. Members can compete for floor time during the discussion. There can be a competition for being a consultee meeting after meeting. Individual members may find themselves competing for the same job while being a member of the same peer group. Competitive feeling may arise at the most unexpected times. Hart-Smith (1985) provides an example of competitiveness during a peer group meeting. At the end of a meeting a member slipped on her new fur coat, which had been inconspicuously folded on a chair in the corner of the room. There was a cry of recognition among several group members and then a chorus of "Sadie, Sadie, Married Lady" broke out. The owner of the coat stood in the group feeling embarrassed and unsure of how to respond. When the song ended, group members departed and the member who was the focus of the joke left feeling uneasy about what had occurred. At the next scheduled meeting several members wanted to process the event, including speculation concerning the competitive feelings that were triggered by a symbol of "having made it." Feelings were explored by all group members and apology made to the group member who had been singled out. The power of being able to talk about such an uncomfortable situation spoke of the maturity of the group and the feeling that, if something feels wrong, it probably ought to be discussed in order to preserve the group.

Diagnosing Group Problems

Groups will experience various bumps in terms of group functioning. If members are continually late, or frequently miss meetings, other members will certainly have feelings about it. If not expressed and processed, these feelings will fester and possibly leak into a consultation by way of hostile comments, and eventually damage the group. If a group member feels that a particular member is often critical of them during the feedback phase of the consultation, it will need to be addressed. In addition, the following could indicate difficulty with group process:

Continual absences of group members
Reluctance on the part of members to present
Extensive socialization interfering with presentations

Lengthy presentation with inadequate time for discussion
Defensiveness exhibited by the consultee
High member dropout rate
Several cancellations of scheduled meetings
Uninspired presentations
Excessive politeness by consultants
Inability to assimilate new members
Inability to let members terminate

Excessive absences can mean that a member or members do not have a significant commitment to the group. If interest in group membership is a fleeting fancy, the member will soon drop out or display poor overall attendance. This may or may not be the fault of the group. Members must be screened initially for their level of commitment and made to understand the importance of attendance, except for unavoidable absences. There is a detrimental effect when members either stop coming to a group altogether or who leave soon after joining a group, except for the very beginning of the group forming. If a member begins to be absent after a record of attendance, it needs to be addressed in case there are either personal or professional reasons at play. The group needs to discuss the norm of group attendance and review the expectations related to attendance. This can also be negotiated at times. For example, a group member who was going out of the country for 6 months negotiated with the group an ability to return to the group when she returned.

Extensive socialization may occur over time as members get more comfortable with one another and begin to care about each other's personal lives. This can be a sign of group cohesion, and so does not portend problems unless the time spent in socializing bleeds into the consultations themselves. This is why it is wise to plan ahead for this opportunity and invite members to come early to enjoy one another's company before the actual meeting begins. In addition, planning a dinner meeting at the beginning and end of each year, or a retreat together, can address the need to connect and meet intimacy needs of members. It bears repeating that if members choose to socialize outside of the meetings, either having lunch together at the workplace or going to a play together, the norm should be that the actual proceedings of the group are not discussed. This limit on social behavior is protective of group functioning.

If presentations begin to be uninspired or too long leaving no time for discussion, it may mean that the consultee is anxious and feeling defensive. It could mean that the consultee is presenting a case that is a show-off sort of case, which has no problem but it is showcasing their talent. This can be particularly galling for the consultants since there is no job to be done, except to flatter the consultee. A good rule is that only problems, dilemmas, and questions are presented. No bragging allowed!

If the presentation is so long that it leaves little time for discussion, it is a good indication that the consultee is hesitant to really get into the meat of the issues. This may not be conscious and, if it becomes a pattern in group, will need to be verbalized by group members. Also, the timekeeper, host, and taskmaster can help with this by reminding people of the time and the next task that needs to be accomplished in the phases.

Excessive politeness during the consultation on the part of the consultants is common during the initial stages of group development. It represents the cautiousness that is common in the early stages before trust is established. Consultants will be hesitant to say anything negative about another member as they do not know if the member or the group can tolerate it. While we all need and seek approval in terms of our work, it is often more valuable to have someone point out a blind spot in terms of our care of patients or relationships with those we work with. The problem is that if too many meeting consist of "you are doing a great job," the meetings will seem flat and unreal, even ingenuous. False reassurance is never very reassuring, even when it comes to providers. Giving feedback that points out areas that the consultee has not looked at, or perhaps made a mistake in, can be provided in a caring and respectful manner. Just like the art of interpretation in psychotherapy, when the therapist confronts a patient's resistance in order to facilitate a breakthrough or insight, it must occur within a caring backdrop. Our best friends can tell us things that we can hear and that we would reject from a stranger or someone who we believe does not have our best interest at hear. If a consultee believes that a consultant is genuinely attempting to be helpful, they are better able to hear difficult feedback. If it is the consultee that is being too polite, such as after stating the question the group goes off on a tangent on another matter that they find interesting, the consultee must speak up and bring the group back to the question. Being too polite might mean that the consultee does not have their needs met.

Handling Personal Events

In the course of being a member of a peer group, often for years at a time, events in one's personal life may impact the peer group. Examples of personal events include pregnancy, infertility, divorce, being fired or promoted, death of a family member, difficulty with an adolescent child, or having a serious illness. Although the priority for a peer group is the consultation work and professional development, personal issues can be accommodated. The impact on the peer group will depend on certain variables such as visibility and timing (Kombrink, 1985). Certain events will be more obvious than others. A pregnancy or illness will become known to group members even if one would prefer to not share them. On the other hand, other issues will be quite invisible and the member will have the option to share it or not. The issue of timing concerns the fact that, in the early stages of group development, sharing personal information ought to be minimized; it will naturally evolve as members feel more connected to one another and develop a natural interest in each others well-being. While some members may choose to share personal events, others choose not to do so. Groups can also decide on the group norm of dealing with personal issues in the group.

While peer groups may begin for the purpose of professional development, they may choose to add the option of asking personal consultation in the group. These may be related to consultations related to parenting, caring for elderly parents, and marriages. The personal and professional may also merge when considering consultations for developing a healthcare practice, proposing a dissertation topic, or considering a job offer. The rich opportunity of hearing the voices of smart and creative peers, who one respects, can be invaluable.

Joining and Leaving Group

As noted previously, there is an optimal number for small group functioning. Therefore, there will be a need at times to consider adding members when members leave the group. Joining any group that has a level of cohesion is always difficult and a peer group is no exception. Methods of recruiting and orienting members have been discussed, but I would add that orientation needs to include a discussion of the philosophy, purposes, and goals of the group with new potential members. Preparing to bring new members aboard can often facilitate this discussion in the group. This process can assist in clarifying these issues and help the group in developing its identity.

The issue of members leaving an existing peer group is important to process. The reasons for the member leaving will of course color the reaction of the remaining members. If it is a premature departure, as a result of the member being dissatisfied with the group, it can be wounding to the group because members may feel either rejected or guilty about how the exiting member was treated. If the departure is the result of a member moving or having a life change that results in them making decisions about time management, the feelings of rejection may be less. It is, however, important to provide enough time in group to discuss all of the feelings that are generated with departures. Some members may feel angry and others sad. It is natural to worry about what the permanent absence of a particular member will mean for the group. This will take time to sort out once the member has left. This is why it is wise to let some time go by before immediately replacing the departing member. The group needs to experience what the new configuration feels like and how successful the group is in achieving group goals.

In this age of the Internet, the online format presents a perfect solution to the issue of a provider who works or lives in a rural area. There are many examples of online groups that solve the problem of group members who have a lot of geography between them. What would seem to be important for such a peer group is a method of screening or matching group members, a clear understanding of how the group is to be structured, and run and clear rules regarding confidentiality.

Summary

Recruit 8–10 members if a start-up group
Decide on where and when to meet, length of meetings
Plan a rotation of hosts and destinations for the year
Decide about refreshments; what will be provided by host
Decide about social time; how much time before meeting
Discuss norms regarding attendance, commitment, absences
Review phases of consultation
Review roles of consultees
Review roles of consultants
Review roles of host, timekeeper, taskmaster
Discuss dinner meeting at beginning and end of year
Discuss idea of a retreat
Begin!

SAMPLE PEER GROUPS

1. Consultation Request: Case Example

Consultee's Question

A group member, a psychotherapist, presented the following clinical case to the group.

"My question is the ethical dilemma of providing support versus psychotherapy in a new patient I have seen three times thus far." The consultee went on with the presentation.

Mrs. S., a 72-year-old married woman was referred to the clinician by her primary care physician. Mrs. S. had been driven to the appointment by her husband, who the patient asked to accompany her into the visit. The patient's husband then described her chief complaint, that of experiencing flashbacks and nightmares and that she began to have a sleep disturbance as a result. After 10 minutes the clinician asked the patient's husband to leave the room and proceeded to conduct the initial interview. It became clear to the consultee that the patient had serious memory problems, as evidenced in the mental status examination. However, both the patient and her husband expressed enthusiasm for returning the following week. In the next two sessions the patient revealed a history of brutal sexual and emotional abuse by her father that she had endured for many years during her childhood. In addition, the patient had been aware of the sexual abuse of her younger sisters and felt extremely guilty about not intervening with her father. The patient would return the following week and report clear improvement in symptoms and affect. Yet the clinician was aware that the patient's early dementia would preclude an ability to conduct psychodynamic psychotherapy and felt uneasy about what she was doing with the patient. Thus she felt the need to consult with the peer group.

Consultants' Response

The consultants asked the consultee for various details about the patient's history and the treatment. Then the group discussed the ethical issue and each weighed in on the matter of charging for psychotherapy. In addition, the consultants shared their experience with patients who, for a variety of reasons, reminded them of this case. It was the group's view that, as a result of the cathartic nature of the sessions, the patient had been able to process emotionally difficult material and, thus, had shown an improvement and that there was no ethical problem. The entire consultation lasted for 30 minutes; the consultee thanked the group and the next presentation was initiated.

Discussion

It was useful for the consultee to present this unusual case to her peers and hear their views about an atypical case. The group was able to frame the work for the consultee in a way that helped address any ethical concerns and let her relax and let the therapy, or whatever name it was to be called, work. If the consultee had not the opportunity to present she might have stewed about the issues for much longer, and perhaps without resolution. Just the process of presenting the case and stating the question had helped the consultee formulate the issues in a way that was useful.

Prologue

The therapist continued to see this patient for a total of eight sessions. At that time the patient and her husband reported marked improvement in symptoms. At that time the therapist initiated ending therapy and making herself available for future contact if needed.

2. Consultation Request: Career Issue

Consultee's Question

"I am pursuing the issue of adoption and, as you know, I am single, so the implications of balancing career and single parenting weigh heavily on me. I want to ask how to configure my practice in order to achieve this balance."

Consultants' Response

The group took turns asking the consultee about how her present practice was configured, how many hours/week she was hoping to work, what childcare arrangements she was thinking of, etc. Other consultants asked the consultee what other professional interest she had beyond the provision of psychotherapy. In fact, the therapist had a longstanding interest in working in the school system, but had never pursued this in her career. Other possible activities were suggested, such as doing group therapy, with a co-therapist, offering to teach a class at a local university, and in a continuing education setting.

Discussion

At the start of the presentation the consultee's anxiety was quite evident. As the group process unfolded and various options were offered by group members, her demeanor became visibly more relaxed. Although no decisions were reached, the consultee expressed her gratitude to the group for opening up potential professional possibilities for her. Hearing from others regarding their strategies for juggling career and family responsibilities was helpful for the consultee. After thanking the members for their ideas, the consultation concluded.

3. Consultation Request: Organizational Issue

Consultee's Question

"I need help figuring out whether to accept a promotion. I have doubts about my ability to do the job and to balance my work with my personal life."

Consultants' Response

The group took turns asking questions that would help to clarify the underlying dilemma faced by the consultee. The group helped the consultee to do a reality check regarding lining up her abilities and the job responsibilities. A group member commented on the natural tendency to feel unsure when faced with career risk taking, or stretching in regard to past role expectations. She shared how anxious she felt before her advancement to teach graduate school, after years of teaching undergraduates at a local college. Other group members tuned into the issue of balancing demands of home and career. Several members shared several strategies for evaluating how to make decisions about the issue of creating and maintaining balance in life. The conversation at times turned to a cleaning service and daycare options. No prescriptions were offered in the group but, rather, sharing of how group members experienced this question, and how they had proceeded in their situation. The group asked the consultee to share in the next group what further thinking had occurred as well as her decision in regard to the promotion.

Discussion

The role of the group was to guide the consultee to ferret out the various issues that were contributing to her confusion about making a career decision. The power of groups are that, by hearing that others have experienced various feelings or thoughts, one often feels inherently less isolated. The power to make the final decision was clearly in the lap of the consultee, and group members refrained from offering an opinion of what she should do in this regard. Not doing so communicated a level of respect for the consultee, in that the group knew that there was no right or wrong conclusion and the fact that the consultee was the best one to weigh the various alternatives and reach a decision.

COMMUNICATION EXERCISES

1. Experiencing a Peer Group

Form a group of four: 1.5 hours.

Participants:

Take turns identifying a clinical case, organizational, or career issue with your group. Take turns. What is your question? Give background information to the group. Conduct a peer consultation for each of the members.

Discussion:

Take turns and share your experiences of presenting and being a consultant in the group.

What was beneficial or helpful?

How could this process be improved?

What is your overall assessment of this process?

Share any experiences in peer groups, and compare and contrast this model with your prior group.

_____

_____

_____

_____

_____

_____

_____

_____

JOURNALING EXERCISES

1. Peer Group Participation

What are your experiences of being in a peer group, either in school or in the clinical setting?

How would describe your personality as a group member?

What thoughts do you have regarding forming or joining a peer group once your academic program is completed?

REFERENCES

Benshoff, J. M. (1994). *Peer consultation as a form of supervision.* Greensboro, NC: ERIC Clearinghouse on Counseling and Student Services.

Borders, L. D. (1991). A systematic approach to peer group supervision. *Journal of Counseling and Development, 69*(3), 248–252.

Briggs, L. A., Heath, J., & Kelly, J. (2005). Peer review for advanced practice nurses: What does it really mean? *AACN Clinical Issues, 16*(1), 3–15.

Counselman, E. F., & Weber, E. (2004). Organizing and maintaining peer supervision groups. *International Journal of Group Psychotherapy, 54*(2), 125–143.

Gavrin, J. (1985). How to present to your peers. In J. Shields, J. Gavrin, V. Hart-Smith, L. Kombrick, J. Kovach, M. Sheehan, et al. *Peer consultation in a group context: A guide for professional nurses.* New York: Springer Publishing Co.

Hart-Smith, V. (1985). How to compete successfully. In J. Shields, J. Gavrin, V. Hart-Smith, L. Kombrink, J. Kovach, M. Sheehan, et al. *Peer consultation in a group context: A guide for professional nurses.* New York: Springer Publishing Co.

Hunt, W., & Issacharoff, A. (1975). History and analysis of a leaderless group of therapists. *American Journal of Psychiatry, 132*(11), 1164–1167.

Kenny, K. J., Baker, L., Lanzon, M., Stephens, L. R., & Yancy, M. (2008). An innovative approach to peer review for the advanced practice nurse—a focus on critical incidents. *Journal of the American Academy of Nurse Practitioners, 20*(7), 376–381.

Kombrink, L. (1985). Why join a peer group? In J. Shields, J. Gavrin, V. Hart-Smith, L. Kombrink, J. Kovach, M. Sheehan, et al. *Peer consultation in a group context: A guide for professional nurses.* New York: Springer Publishing Co.

Kovach, J. S. (1985). What is peer consultation in a group context? In J. Shields, J. Gavrin, V. Hart-Smith, L. Kombrink, J. Kovach, M. Sheehan, et al. (1985). *Peer consultation in a group context: A guide for professional nurses.* New York: Springer Publishing Co.

Lassiter, P. S., Napolitano, L., Culbreth, J. R., & Ng, K. (2008). Developing multicultural competence using the structured peer group supervision model. *Counselor Education and Supervision, 47*(3), 164–178.

Phelan, A. M., Barlow, C. A., & Iversen, S. (2006). Occasioning learning in the workplace: The case of interprofessional peer collaboration. *Journal of Interprofessional Care, 20*(4), 415–424.

Sheehan, M. (1985). How to confront successfully. In J. Shields, J. Gavrin, V. Hart-Smith, L. Kombrink, J. Kovach, M. Sheehan, et al. *Peer consultation in a group context: A guide for professional nurses.* New York: Springer Publishing Co.

Sheilds, J., Garvrin, J., Hart-Smith, V., Kombrink, L., Kovach, J. Sheehan, M., et al. (1985). *Peer consultation in a group context: A guide for professional nurses.* New York: Springer Publishing Co.

Thomasgard, M., Warfield, J., & Williams, R. (2004). Improving communication between health and infant mental health professionals utilizing ongoing collaborative peer supervision groups. *Infant Mental Health Journal, 25*(3), 194–218.

Tisdall, M., & O'Donoghue, K. (2003). A facilitated peer group supervision model for practitioners. In K. McMaster, & A. Wells (Eds.). *Innovative approaches to stopping family violence* (pp. 221–232). Wellington, New Zealand: Steele Roberts.

Zagata, K. How to respond to peers. In J. Shields, J. Garvrin, V. Hart-Smith, L. Kombrink, J. Kovach, M. Sheehan, et al. (1985). *Peer consultation in a group context: A guide for professional nurses.* New York: Springer Publishing Co.

Index

Page numbers followed by *b*, *f*, or *t* indicate material in boxes, figures, or tables, respectively.